BATHING

FOR HEALTH, BEAUTY & RELAXATION

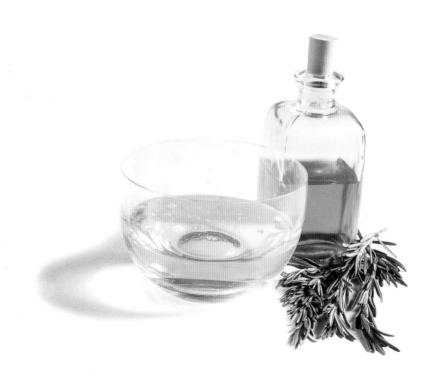

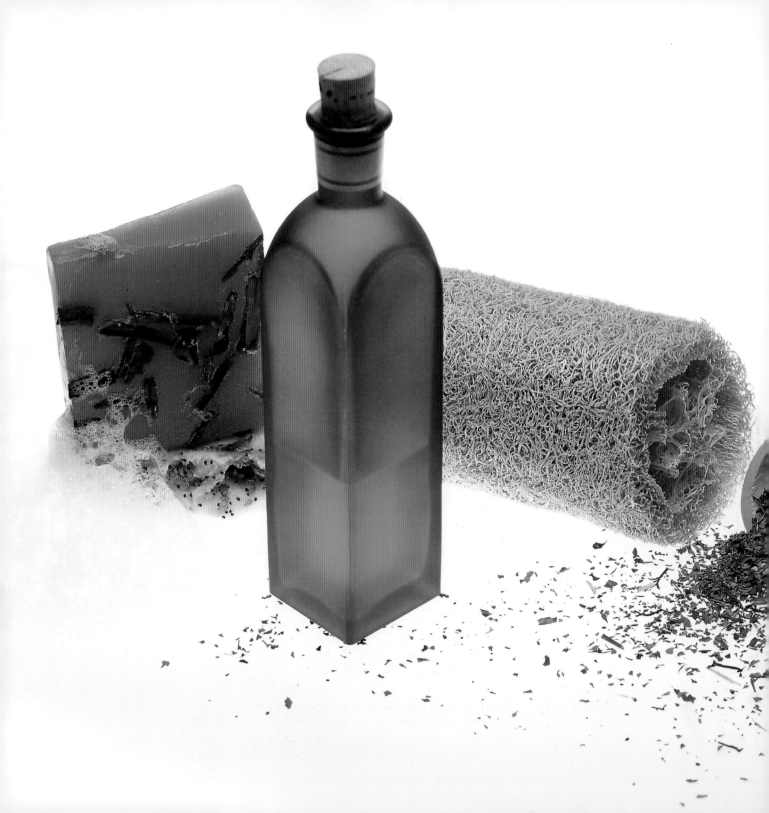

BATHING

FOR HEALTH, BEAUTY & RELAXATION

EVA GIZOWSKA

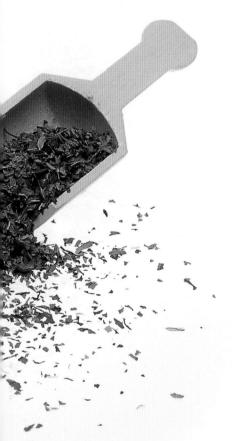

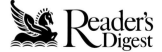

PUBLISHED BY THE READER'S DIGEST ASSOCIATION LIMITED

London • New York • Sydney • Cape Town • Montreal

A READER'S DIGEST BOOK

Published by

The Reader's Digest Association Limited

11 Westferry Circus

Canary Wharf

London

E14 4HE

Cataloguing in Publication Data is available from
the British Library

ISBN 0 276 42396 8

A QUARTO BOOK

Copyright © 1998 Quarto Publishing plc

Designed and edited by Quarto Publishing plc

The Old Brewery

6 Blundell Street

London N7 9BH

Senior Project Editor: **Gerrie Purcell**

Text Editors: **Mary Senechal, Hilary Sagar, Eric Chaline**

Senior Art Editor: **Penny Cobb**

Designers: **Ruth Hope, Luise Roberts**

Picture Researcher: **Christine Lalla**

Photographer: **Will White**

3-D Photo-Illustration: **Mandy Pritty**

Illustrator: **Janice Nicolson**

Art Director: **Moira Clinch**

Publisher: **Marion Hasson**

Typeset in Great Britain by
Central Southern Typesetters, Eastbourne
Manufactured by Bright Arts (Singapore) Pte Ltd
Printed in China by Leefung-Asco Printers Ltd

TO THE READER

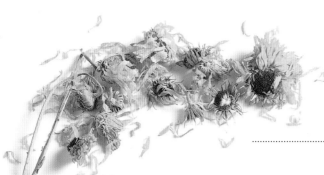

CONTENTS

....

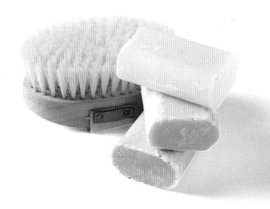

$\mathcal{I}$NTRODUCTION

TO THINK OF BATHING solely in terms of cleansing the body is to ignore the many ways in which this daily ritual can enhance your well-being. Bathing offers a multitude of benefits. It can be a therapeutic, sensual, calming, invigorating, or uplifting experience. Not sure where to start? Let this book point you in the right direction.

The book begins with the basics — from the benefits of regular skin brushing through advice on the right kind of soap or body lotion. Individual sections show how bathing can help you feel healthier and happier. *Cleansing Baths* tells you how to use saunas, steam baths and detoxifying herbs. *Conditioning Baths* lets you into the secrets of therapeutic treatments such as mineral, mud and seaweed baths. *Relaxing Baths* shows you how bathing can help you unwind mentally and physically. If you are troubled by a specific physical complaint, such as aching muscles, rheumatism or psoriasis, *Bathing for Well-Being* has advice on beneficial therapies. For an eye-opening tonic, turn to *Invigorating Baths* for ingredients and bathing techniques to boost energy. Special features explain how bathing rituals and traditions have changed throughout the ages.

The emphasis throughout the book is on natural ingredients and products such as herbs, plants, flowers and essential oils. These are readily obtainable from health food shops and other sources. You can use most of the remedies, therapies and other water treatments in your own bathroom. However, if you want to treat yourself to a visit to a spa, find inspiration in the section on premier spas in North America, Europe and throughout the world.

E. Gizowska

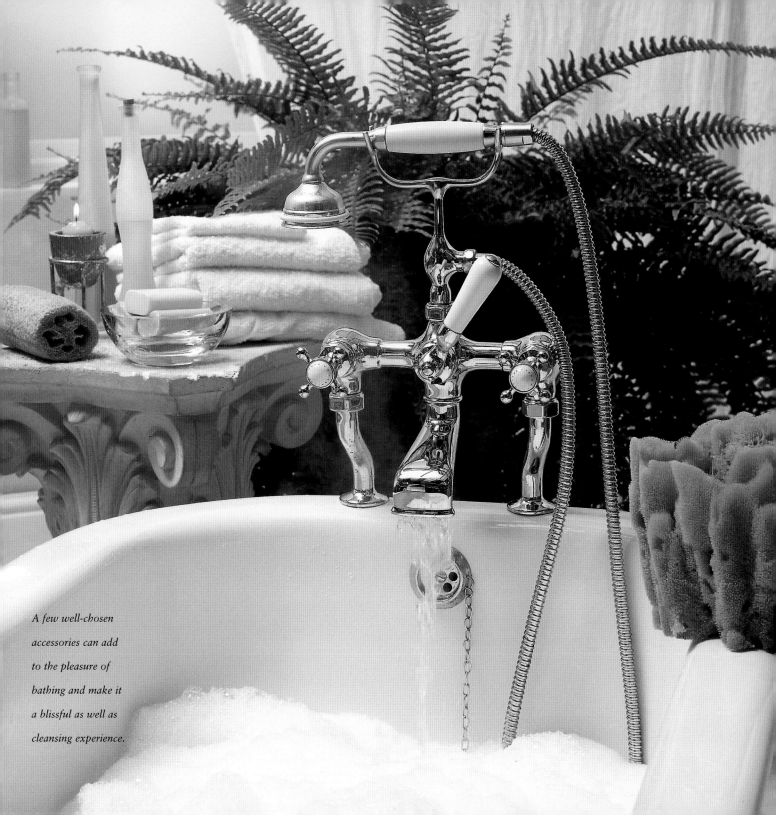

A few well-chosen accessories can add to the pleasure of bathing and make it a blissful as well as cleansing experience.

A BRIEF HISTORY OF BATHING

TAKING A BATH OR SHOWER seems a modern concept, but baths have been around since at least 2000 BC — as we know from artifacts found in the Indus Valley, Asia. In Greece at the time of Homer (c. 8th century BC), preparing a hot, scented bath for a guest was as much a mark of hospitality as offering food and drink. The ancient Egyptians considered bathing to be essential to their health and well-being and often used aromatic oils and other fragrances in their baths. They were also the first to make soap, from the soapwort plant. However, the greatest advances in bathing were made by the Romans.

Mixed public baths that remained in some 16th-century European cities were deemed a health risk.

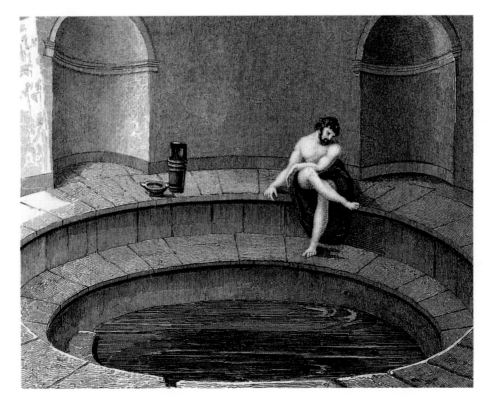

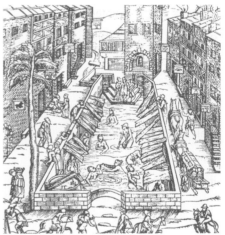

A small Greek or Roman bathhouse, depicted on a vase. Bathing was important to both these ancient cultures, which used scented baths for personal health and enjoyment, and as a means of welcoming guests.

Roman Baths

To the ancient Romans, bathing was an integral part of their daily lives. After exercise in the gymnasium at the public baths, or thermae, the Roman would first take a cool shower in the frigidarium — a vast, vaulted room at the centre of the baths. This was followed by a massage and a succession of warm and hot baths (in the tepidarium and caldarium). Then it was back to the frigidarium for a final cold shower and an invigorating rub-down. The Romans understood the therapeutic benefits of water, and physicians regularly prescribed cold-water cures, sweating treatments and vapours for particular illnesses. The Romans also liked to bathe in scented water and anoint their bodies with aromatic oils. The Emperor Caligula, notorious for his cruelty, is said to have enjoyed relaxing in a rosewater bath.

By the end of the 4th century AD, the city of Rome had 856 public baths. Wherever the Romans conquered they installed their spectacular baths. Today, these legacies of the Roman Empire can be seen in various places in Europe, such as Bath in England and Aix-les-Bains in France.

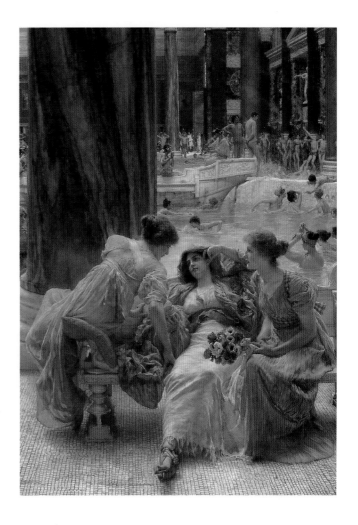

A Return to Grime

The overthrow of the Roman Empire in the 5th century, and the growth of Christianity, brought about a dramatic change in attitudes towards bathing. The barbarian tribes who conquered Rome found scented baths and the obsession with cleanliness incomprehensible. In addition the Church disapproved of the decadence of the elaborate Roman bathing rituals. With bathhouses no longer deemed acceptable, many of the technologies instigated by the Romans disappeared. Europe was plunged back into its former grimy ways, and it wasn't until the 18th century that bathing became popular again.

The delights of Roman bathing inspired this idyllic portrayal of the Baths of Caracalla by Sir Lawrence Alma-Tadema.

Bathing Revival

The bathing revival was prompted by the re-emergence of the interest in classical spas and the use of water as a health aid. Spas were established in many locations in Europe and North America, and it became the height of fashion to visit them. People flocked to Wiesbaden in Germany to sip the mineral water and submerge themselves in mud baths. In England, healing waters put towns such as Tunbridge Wells, Malvern, Epsom and Bath on the 19th-century tourist map. In the United States, stagecoaches carried thousands of health-seekers to resorts such as Boyes Hot Springs in California and the Hot Springs in Arkansas.

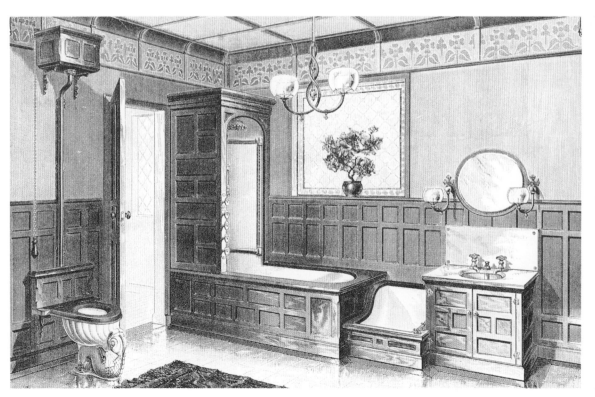

Gettysburg Springs in Pennsylvania in the 19th century. Thousands flocked to spas in the United States and Europe in a movement motivated by fashion as well as health.

A prestigious early 20th-century bathroom included a porcelain bath, copper shower and 'needle sprays', a 'seat and foot' bath and a toilet.

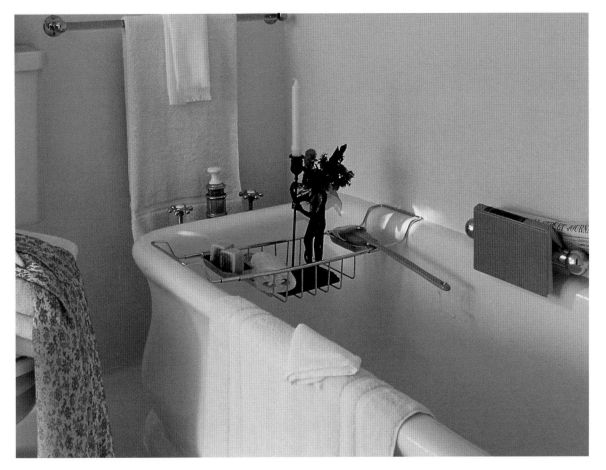

As ownership of bathrooms grew during the 20th century, cast-iron baths replaced their portable tin and copper predecessors. Ornate bathrooms gave way to clinical designs which emphasised the hygienic functions of the room.

Home Bathrooms

The discovery that germs spread disease transformed attitudes to bathing. People began washing more and this increased demand for bathing facilities. Tin and copper hip baths (small portable baths) were gradually replaced by full-size cast-iron baths — the first to be installed in the White House arrived in 1851. The Victorians found the idea of devoting one room exclusively to bathing self-indulgent, but by the end of the 19th century owning a bathroom had became a status symbol. By the 1930s, even lower-income groups began to have bathrooms. With the possibility of luxuriating in one's own bathroom came a renewed association of cleanliness and health with the pampering and pleasurable aspects of bathing.

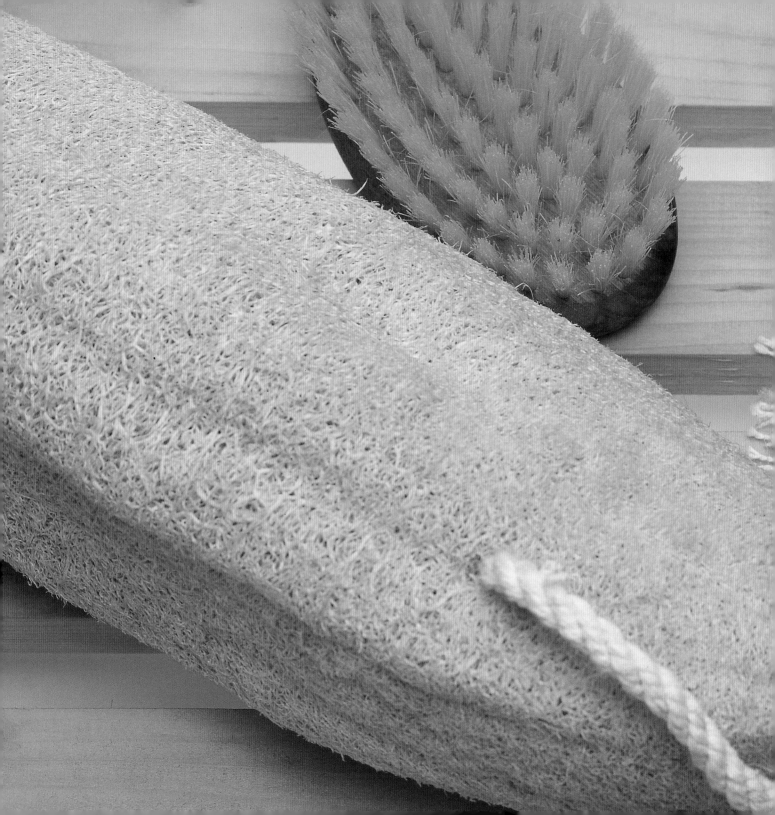

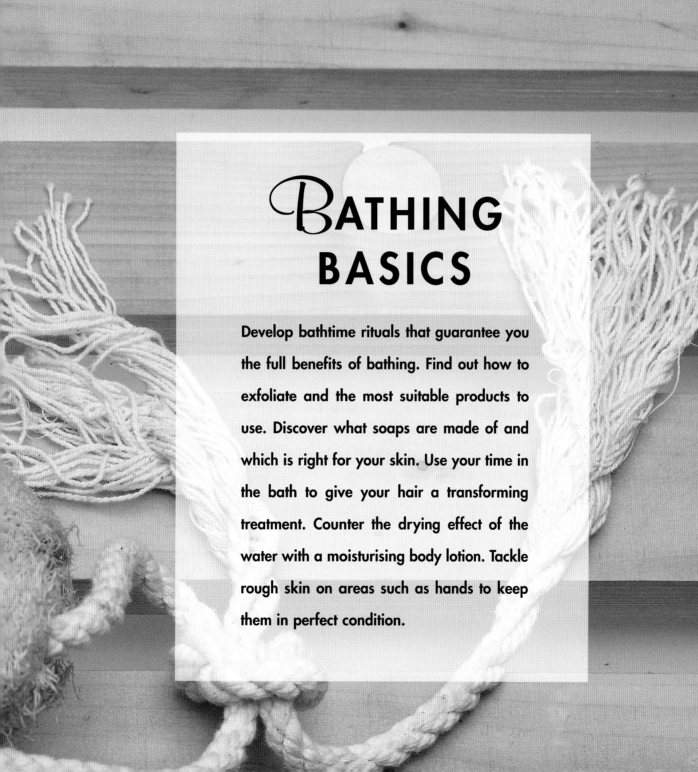

Bathing Basics

Develop bathtime rituals that guarantee you the full benefits of bathing. Find out how to exfoliate and the most suitable products to use. Discover what soaps are made of and which is right for your skin. Use your time in the bath to give your hair a transforming treatment. Counter the drying effect of the water with a moisturising body lotion. Tackle rough skin on areas such as hands to keep them in perfect condition.

Skin brushing

Simple techniques, such as scrubbing or brushing your skin before you jump into the bath or shower, not only feel good but are immensely beneficial.

Regular exfoliation helps to remove dead particles, leaving the skin softer and smoother. The friction also boosts circulation and unclogs blocked pores, so that the skin looks fresher.

The process of skin renewal can be slowed down by factors that include stress, the action of hormones, changes in temperature and climate, and ageing. When the regeneration of skin cells takes longer, there is an increased build-up of dry, dull-looking skin, especially on the areas where blood circulation is poorest, such as heels, elbows and knees (see also Special-care zones, pages 22–3).

Facial Exfoliators

Some of the most popular facial exfoliators are chemical products containing AHAs (alpha hydroxy acids); naturally occurring substances derived from milk, sugar cane and fruits, which have a mild exfoliant effect. Physical exfoliators, similar to those used on the body, are equally effective. Use facial exfoliators once a week if your skin is dry, two or three times a week if your skin is oily.

There are several ways to exfoliate skin. You can do it through vigorous brushing with a body brush, or scrubber, scrub glove or mitt. Or you can use exfoliating creams and gels.

Body Brushing

Body brushing is best done every morning. It is a great way to boost circulation and wake yourself up. Use a soft hand brush or an abrasive glove or mitt to massage your arms, stomach, buttocks, thighs and legs gently and briskly. A longer brush or scrubber makes it easier to reach your back.

Exfoliating Creams and Gels

Exfoliators come in two varieties; so-called physical exfoliators, based on natural, mildly abrasive ingredients (such as oatmeal, wheat germ, rice grains or jojoba — a natural wax derivative), and the chemical creams and gels produced by the major cosmetic companies. Both types are pleasant and easy to use. Apply them directly to your skin, or

Skin brushing can be done wet or dry. Use exfoliating cream for a thorough scrub, or soap if you want lather. A natural sponge gives a gentle rub and pumice stones are for feet.

mix them with a little water on the palm of your hand and massage lightly into the skin. Rinse off the lotion thoroughly with warm water.

Caution Do not exfoliate if you are currently suffering from any skin irritation or allergies. Avoid moles and varicose veins.

Body Scrub Equipment

Scrubbing tools come in all shapes and sizes. Certain tools are best used on particular parts of the body. Always use soft fibres on delicate skin areas.

Body scrubber (loofah) made from the fibrous tissues of the dishcloth gourd (*Luffa*). Apply to wet skin. After use, rinse and hang to dry. Replace frequently.

Long-handled back brush for hard-to-reach parts of your back. Use wet or dry. Rub your palm against the bristles to check they are not too stiff.

Smaller body brushes for scrubbing legs and arms.

Natural sponge is formed from sea organisms. Especially suitable for sensitive skins.

Pumice is a light, porous, very hard piece of volcanic rock for exfoliating the skin on your feet.

Hemp glove as an alternative to the body brush, made from the tough fibres of the hemp plant. Use dry or with exfoliator cream or gel.

Sisal body scrub mitt made from cactus fibres which give it its abrasive surface; good for a brisk rub.

Brush firmly but not hard towards your heart; up the legs and arms, up over the abdomen and down from the shoulder blades to the chest.

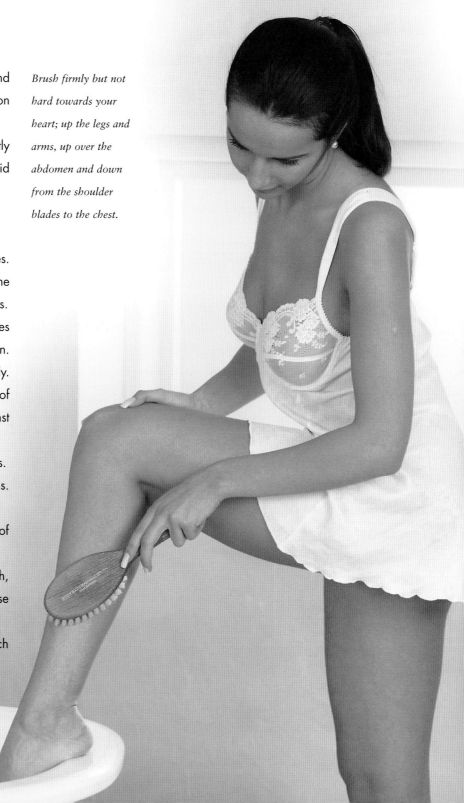

Soaps and gels

Plain and functional, scented and elaborate — soaps and gels are the chief personal cleansers in any bathroom. It is important to understand their formulations because they effect the health of your skin.

The main ingredient of most soaps is tallow, a substance derived from animal fats, which is mixed with caustic soda and water. Hard fats create firm, long-lasting soap. Softer fats produce creamier, milder soaps, which dissolve more readily.

Not all soaps contain animal by-products. Synthetic soaps are manufactured from detergents and mineral oils. Vegetable soaps contain oils such as olive, sunflower or jojoba. Shower gels and bubble baths are closer in formulation to shampoos. They contain a higher percentage of chemicals and detergents to increase their lather, and often include more fragrance and colourants.

Too Much of a Good Thing?

Although soaps and gels are effective cleansers, they can be harsh to the skin, stripping it of oils and upsetting the natural pH (or acid/alkaline) balance. In order to protect your skin, choose formulations with the mildest ingredients (see the box right). Alternatively, make your own soap from one of the recipes on page 93.

Choosing Your Cleanser

For dry skins

Creamy soaps with a rich texture, containing ingredients such as almond, jojoba, avocado and olive oils.

For oily skins

Gels and soaps containing citrus or fruit essential oils.

For most skin types

Glycerine soaps.

For sensitive skins

Vegetable-based or glycerine soaps containing vitamin E and aloe vera. Also, the mild soaps specifically developed for delicate skin types.

To smooth the skin and boost circulation

Exfoliating soaps, containing oats, bran and other seeds and plant fibres.

Traditional varieties are 'triple-milled' (repeatedly ground and mixed) to improve the consistency of texture and colour. These soaps are more expensive than mass-produced brands, but they do not crack or disintegrate so easily. Triple-milling and natural ingredients produce some of the finest but also the most highly priced soaps.

Read a soap label and you will probably see linoleic, lauric or palmitic acid among the ingredients. They are the key to the qualities you can expect to find in the soap.

How readily soap lathers and how well it cleanses or conditions are determined by which of these fatty acids predominates in the base fat. For example, palm oil is high in palmitic acid, which increases hardness. Lauric acid, found in coconut oil, makes soap firm and cleansing, with a rich lather.

Soaps labeled 'super-fatted' are enriched with additional oil — such as coconut, avocado or peach kernel — to soothe and moisturise the skin. Some soaps incorporate natural ingredients, such as oats and wheat germ, to increase their skin-smoothing properties. Others contain exfoliating grains and plant fibres — luffa, bran, millet seeds and seaweed, for example. Soaps can be made

of glycerine (glycerol), an odourless, viscous liquid which can be manufactured from animal or plant materials. It is a natural humectant (moisturiser), which is mild and nourishing to the skin.

Liquid soap is produced by the same method as traditional soaps, but synthetics are added to make it fluid. It can be a useful, hygienic option.

Some of these glycerine soaps have grains and parts of herbs added to them to enhance the cleansing and exfoliating properties.

Healthy and beautiful hair

Having glossy, healthy, clean hair makes us feel good and adds to an overall look of being well-groomed. But we have to look after our hair with good-quality products suited to our hair type to get the best results.

▼ *Check the label when choosing a 'natural' hair care product to gauge how beneficial the natural ingredients may be.*

Modern shampoos are often too good at keeping hair clean. Used in excess, they not only strip the hair of dirt but can upset the balance of naturally occurring oils. Dry hair can become more brittle, and greasy hair can become even more oily as the scalp produces additional oil to compensate. Many hair preparations contain a high percentage of alcohol, which has a very drying effect; silicones, which cling to the hair shaft and eventually weaken it, and chemical dyes, which can in time cause structural damage. Stress, sickness, poor diet and drug treatment can also make hair thinner and reduce its lustre.

Which Shampoo?

Protein shampoos
are also formulated to give the hair more body. The proteins may be synthetic or derived from natural sources, such as soya, gelatin or milk. The synthetic type can contain a high percentage of chemicals.

Rich, creamy nut or vegetable-oil shampoos
(based on coconut, avocado or jojoba) are beneficial for dry hair.

Citrus blends
such as lemon or lime are good for greasy hair. They help to remove oil without leaving hair limp.

Herbal shampoos
can be attractive, but are only therapeutic if the type and quantity of natural ingredients is stated.

Balsams
contain the resins from plants or trees. Their gluey texture coats the hair shaft and helps to make hair look thicker.

Head Massage

A daily 5–10 minute massage can promote blood flow to the scalp and enhance the quality of your hair.

1 *Using your fingertips, work over the surface of the scalp, temples and back of head, applying pressure in circular movements.*

2 *Gently pull at the roots, all over your head, to stimulate the hair follicles.*

3 *Tap the scalp gently with a clenched fist.*

4 *Apply pressure with your fingers to the points shown below. Press each point to the count of three.*

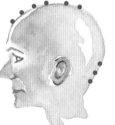

Revitalising pressure points

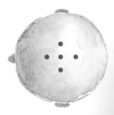

Calming pressure points

- **Normal hair** is strong, easy to style and glossy.
- **Dry hair** appears brittle and tends to become fluffy. Sometimes it is greasy at the scalp.
- **Oily hair** becomes greasy very quickly and can look limp. Fine, 'baby' hair is most subject to oiliness.

A shower is good for shampooing, but try to apply conditioner during a bath, when the warm, steamy atmosphere aids absorption.

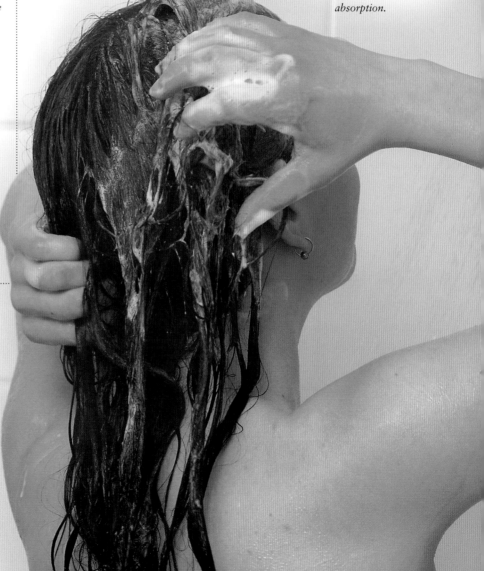

A New Head of Hair

Fortunately hair is constantly renewing itself. Hair grows about 1.25cm (½in) a month and has a lifespan of four to five years. So no matter what condition your hair is in now, by treating it with care you can begin growing a healthy head of hair.

Analysing your hair Start by assessing the overall condition of your hair. This determines the type of product you should choose.

Body moisturisers

Dryness makes the skin taut and dull. Body lotions, creams and gels renew moisture and suppleness.

Rough, flaky skin occurs whenever the moisture levels in the top layer of the skin become depleted. Stress, poor diet, pollution and long hours spent in a centrally heated environment can be the cause. The most effective antidote is to apply body moisturiser every day, after your bath or shower.

Which Moisturiser?

Body moisturisers are available in a variety of formulations. Heavy creams, which are best suited for very dry skin, have a richer texture than lotions and gels. They contain more oil than water. The lighter creams and lotions contain more water than oil and are therefore more fluid. Gels are also predominantly water-based, but are made with natural emollient resins and gums instead of oil. They are most suitable for normal to oily skins.

The primary characteristic of a moisturiser is determined by the oils it contains. Vegetable oils, such as olive, wheat germ, sesame and safflower, are nourishing and rich, so they are often used in dry skin creams. Almond, peach, apricot, jojoba, avocado and grapeseed oils are finer. They make

Damp and warm skin absorbs moisturisers more readily, so the best time to apply them is immediately after bathing. Choose a product suitable for your skin type and smooth it in well.

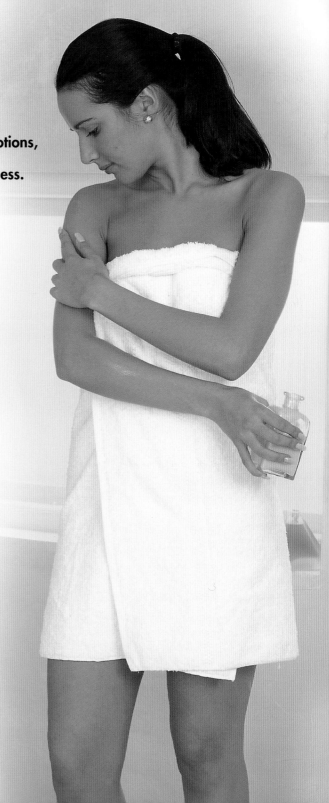

a good base for some of the lighter creams and lotions, and are suitable for normal to dry skins. These oils also make wonderful body lotions in their own right. Massage them into your skin after a hot bath. They will leave your skin oily so they are best applied last thing at night.

Quality Checks

Other oils that you might encounter in body lotions are those made from animal fats, such as lanolin (from sheep), which is thick and waxy, and mineral oils, derived from petroleum. Mineral oils are the cheapest oils to produce, and also the least effective. Instead of being absorbed, they form a greasy layer on the skin. Avoid them if your skin is sensitive, because they frequently cause irritation.

Most moisturisers have a shelf life of 12–18 months. Check the use-by date. Discard the product if it turns cloudy or you notice a marked difference in its smell. Use natural products within 3–6 months.

There is no need to spend a fortune on products to keep your skin in peak condition — you can make your own. Turn to the recipe for Floral Body Oil on page 94.

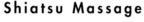

Shiatsu Massage

Shiatsu is Japanese for 'finger pressure' and describes a form of massage equivalent to acupressure. Its purpose is to stimulate the flow of energy (known as chi) around the body and so relieve the blockages that can cause physical and emotional problems. The energy travels along channels (or meridians) dotted with pressure points, known as tsubos, and massaging these boosts the energy flow. Apply your chosen oil over your entire body, using circular movements. Then press each tsubo firmly with your finger and hold for a few seconds.

The points on the arms can help with digestion. Those on the back can help to release tension and promote glowing skin. Points on the front improve circulation, tone the pelvic area and help regulate your appetite. Massaging leg points eases muscle stiffness.

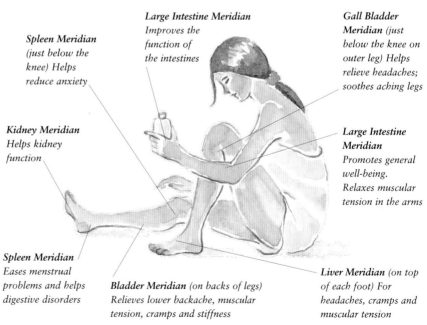

Spleen Meridian *(just below the knee) Helps reduce anxiety*

Kidney Meridian *Helps kidney function*

Spleen Meridian *Eases menstrual problems and helps digestive disorders*

Large Intestine Meridian *Improves the function of the intestines*

Bladder Meridian *(on backs of legs) Relieves lower backache, muscular tension, cramps and stiffness*

Gall Bladder Meridian *(just below the knee on outer leg) Helps relieve headaches; soothes aching legs*

Large Intestine Meridian *Promotes general well-being. Relaxes muscular tension in the arms*

Liver Meridian *(on top of each foot) For headaches, cramps and muscular tension*

Special-care zones

Hands, elbows, knees and feet need extra attention but are often overlooked. Here are some tips for taking good care of them.

Your hands work hard and are on show, so it's important that they look good; smooth and supple, with clean, well-shaped nails. Pay particular attention to your hands as you get older. Wrinkled, gnarled hands make you seem older than you are. For hands to be proud of, adopt the following tactics:

- Moisturise your hands regularly throughout the day (see recipe for Olive Oil Hand Conditioner, page 91). For additional intensive treatment, apply moisturiser at bedtime and sleep in a pair of white cotton gloves. Your hands will feel silky and smooth in the morning.

- Cut your nails regularly and apply softening wheat germ, avocado, or almond oil to condition them and help you push the cuticles back.
- If you have dry, rough patches, exfoliate regularly (see Skin brushing, pages 14–15), using a suitable exfoliator. Then add a few drops of softening oil, such as almond or sesame, to warm water, and soak your hands in it for a few minutes. Dry your hands gently and apply some moisturising hand cream.
- Massage your hands to boost circulation and loosen sore areas. First massage your palm and the back of your hand with fingers and thumb. Then work on your fingers, in a gentle circular motion, pulling slightly from the base of each finger.
- Protect the back of your hands with sunscreen when exposed to the sun.

Elbows and Knees

If your elbows and knees are dry and scaly, exfoliate regularly — with coarse sea salt, for example — and apply freshly squeezed lemon juice, or a halved lemon, to soften the skin. Moisturise after bathing.

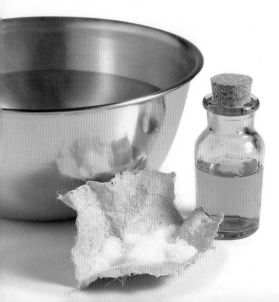

◀ Almond oil in warm water softens hands, while sea salt can help you exfoliate rough skin from your elbows and knees.

Feet

It's easy to forget your feet — yet they have to carry your entire body weight. It's no wonder that these extremities exhibit signs of strain.

- Treat your feet as kindly as your hands by following the same treatments.
- Exfoliate regularly to eliminate dry skin.
- Refresh your feet with a home foot spa. Place them in a bowl of hot water containing a cupful of apple cider vinegar or some Epsom salts. Add a few drops of peppermint essential oil, diluted in massage base oil.
- See the recipe on page 91 for a refreshing foot rub lotion made with calendula petals.

Home Facial

There is probably more mystique surrounding the facial than any other salon treatment — but don't be discouraged by sophisticated-sounding techniques. Your home facial is a simple procedure of cleansing, toning and moisturising, followed by a face mask. Note that men as much as women can benefit from some or all of this treatment, if only to cleanse away everyday grime and tone the skin, in addition to the pleasure to be had from being pampered.

The most crucial factor for a facial is to use the correct products for your skin. A deep-cleansing mask for oily skin will not help a dry, sensitive complexion, which needs intensive moisturising. There is no need to rub and scrub during the course of the treatment. Use a light massaging action to apply and remove each product.

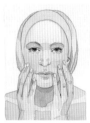

1 *Begin by cleansing. Massage the chosen cleanser onto your skin with your fingertips, and remove with cotton wool pads. These are easier to use than regular cotton wool pulled from a roll. Repeat cleansing until the pad is clean.*

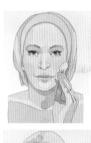

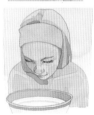

2 *Apply toner to remove any excess cleanser. Choose a toner which is only mildly astringent.*

3 *Steam your face over a bowl or sink of hot water to open the pores. Don't overdo it — too much steaming can damage the tiny blood vessels under your skin. Three to five minutes is long enough. Keep your face at least 15cm (6in) from the water. If you have blackheads, gently squeeze them to the surface after steaming, using a clean tissue.*

4 *Rinse your face with cool water and pat dry. Apply a mask. Try a light gel mask if your skin feels dry, or a heavier clay mask if it is oily. Leave the face mask on for 3–5 minutes. Rinse off with warm water. Then rinse with cool water.*

5 *Apply moisturiser.*

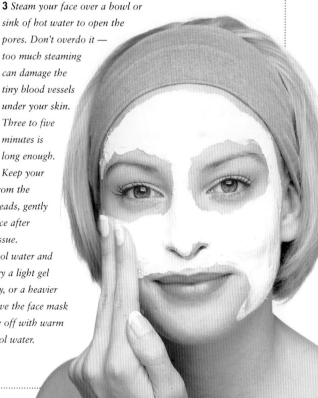

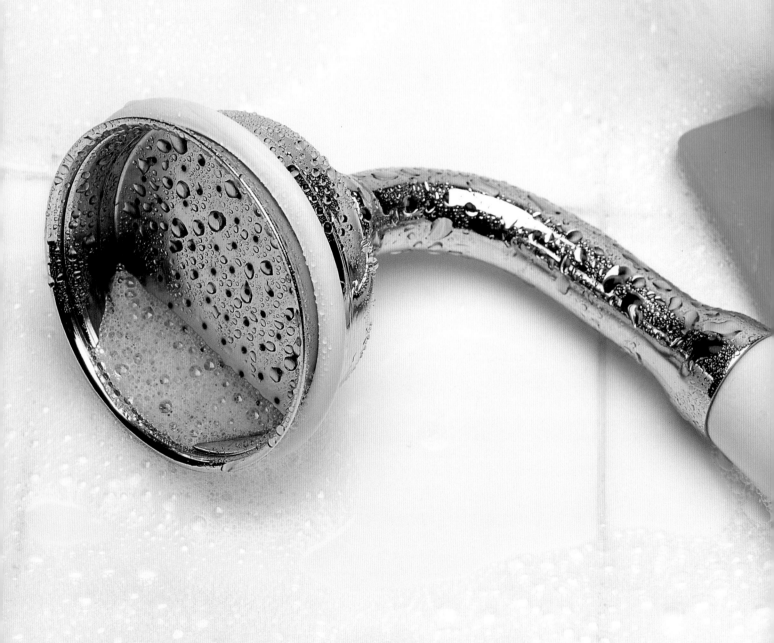

CLEANSING BATHS

Bathing can clean your skin but that is not the same as feeling cleansed from within. Take your bathing one step further by visiting a sauna or steam room — or recreate their effects in your own bathroom. Sweating helps expel toxins through the pores of the skin. Or try a therapeutic herbal bath. Certain herbs also stimulate perspiration, boost metabolism and promote thorough cleansing.

Deep-cleansing saunas

Sweating it out in the sauna is one of the simplest and most effective ways to cleanse your body from within. Carrying impurities out of your system by natural means, a sauna has benefits for your health, appearance and well-being.

The intense dry heat of the sauna causes the blood vessels to expand and promote sweating, which is an excellent inner body cleanser. Although most of your sweat is water, about 10–30 per cent consists of chemical toxins acquired through stress, pollution or diet. Besides eliminating excess wastes, sweating in the sauna speeds your metabolism, boosts your immune system, has a therapeutic effect on aching muscles and joints, and helps to clear your skin of impurities, leaving it soft and radiant. It can also counteract tiredness and 'toxic' headaches.

To obtain maximum benefit, have a sauna at least once a week. After exercise is a good time, because the heat can flush out lactic acid from your muscles and ward off stiffness. Schedule a session for when you are not rushed. Part of the therapeutic value of a sauna is the opportunity to unwind.

The heat in a sauna comes from a stove that creates a temperature of around 80°C (176°F). Only stay in the sauna for as long as you feel comfortable. Five to ten minutes is usually enough. If you can face it, and you are in good health, it is invigorating to jump into a cold shower afterwards. If that sounds drastic, take a warm shower instead.

Scandinavian Style

The concept of the sauna, with its hallmark wooden interior, benches to relax on and branches of fragrant birch leaves to stimulate the circulation, is typically Scandinavian. In Finland there are nearly as many saunas as there are people. On weekends, families and friends regularly head into the country to stay in wooden chalets, complete with sauna, tucked away in acres of lush forest, usually near a river or lake. The Finns think nothing of having a sauna and then jumping into the icy water — or in wintertime, rolling around in the snow.

◄ Take a cool shower after each session in the sauna, and drink lots of water to prevent dehydration. A banana can help to replace the loss of potassium in perspiration, which may cause feelings of weakness.

Taking a Sauna

- *Do not have a sauna immediately after eating. Drink plenty of water during and after a session*
- *Always take a hot shower beforehand*
- *Check the temperature does not exceed 80°C (176°F)*
- *Leave the sauna immediately if you start to feel dizzy*
- *Wear no more than a towel or swimsuit. Remove all jewellery and your watch — the metal will become very hot*
- *Do not spend longer than 5–10 minutes at a time in the sauna. Take a cool shower and rest between sessions*
- *Hot air rises, so sit on the lower benches first. As you become accustomed to the heat, you can move to the higher ones*
- *Take a cool shower when you come out, and rest for at least 30 minutes*
- *Drink water and eat a banana to help replace lost potassium*

Caution *Do not take a sauna if you have any of the following conditions:*
- *Heart disease • Asthma • Respiratory problems*
- *Hypertension • Epilepsy • If you feel you are coming down with an illness • If you have a cold or flu • If you have diabetes, always check with your doctor on the advisability of a sauna • If you are pregnant, check advisability with your doctor, and never take a sauna in the last months of pregnancy — it can induce labour*

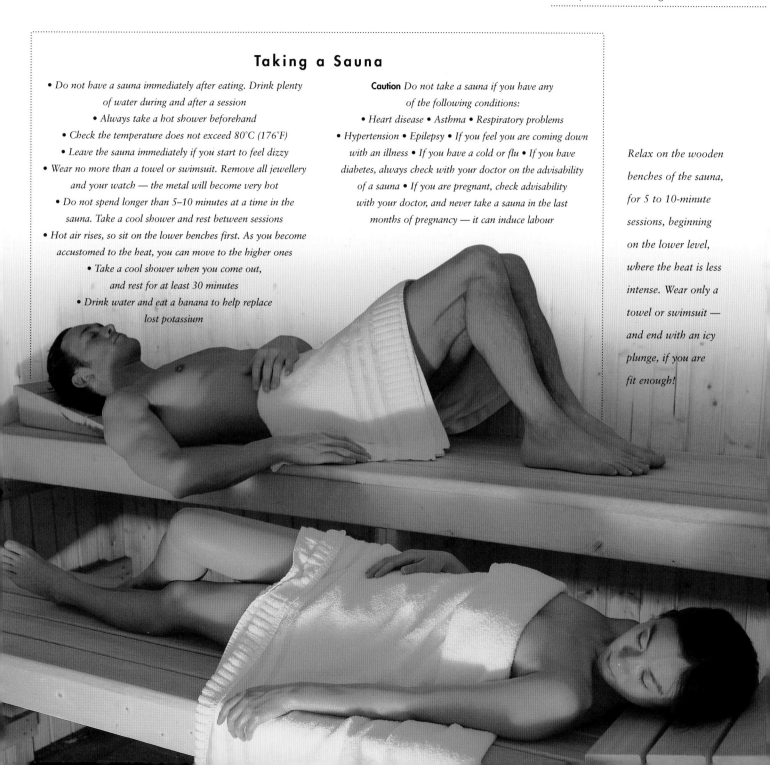

Relax on the wooden benches of the sauna, for 5 to 10-minute sessions, beginning on the lower level, where the heat is less intense. Wear only a towel or swimsuit — and end with an icy plunge, if you are fit enough!

Purifying steam

You can reproduce the stimulating effects of a steam room at home in your own bathroom. Do not be discouraged by the prospect of a cold shower — it will be welcome after the heat of the steam, and the experience will leave you feeling refreshed and purified.

Most health clubs, gyms and spas have steam rooms or cabinets as well as saunas. They work in a similar way to saunas, but the heat is generated differently. Steam room heat is known as wet heat, because it is produced by boiling water. Water boils at 100°C (212°F), which means that the heat in a steam room is intense. Typical Turkish steam rooms often operate at 120–140°C (248–284°F)! The steam is gradually diffused throughout the room to create a hot, humid

Care of Face

Combine your home steam bath with a pore-cleansing facial. Wash your face gently before you steam. At the end of your bath, spray your face with cool water, pat dry and apply a face mask, suitable for your skin type. The steam is less concentrated than when you steam your face directly over hot water, but do not expose oily skin for more than 10 minutes or dry skin for more than five. Protect your face with a face flannel moistened with water infused with your favourite herb or essential oil.

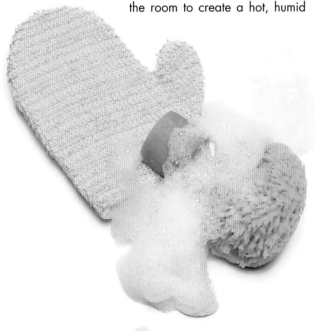

environment which makes you perspire. The heat causes blood vessels to dilate, which increases the rate of blood circulation. Just as with saunas, the aim of a steam room is to make you sweat profusely, and so eliminate toxins from your system.

Steam or Sauna?

Whether you opt for a sauna or steam treatment is a matter of personal preference — the benefits are virtually the same. Do not take a steam bath if you

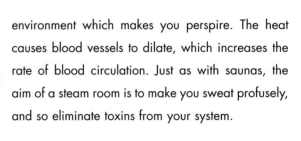

◀ *After your steam session, wash grime and dead skin cells away under a warm shower, using an abrasive sisal mitt or softer natural sponge and vegetable soap.*

Your Own Steam Room

1 *Turn on your shower at the highest temperature. Close all of the doors and windows. The room will begin to fill with steam within about 10 minutes*
2 *Fill a cheesecloth or muslin bag with herbs, such as camomile, lime blossom or elderflowers, and hang it under the running water*
3 *Turn the water off and sit in the steam-filled bathroom for about 10 minutes*
4 *Use the time to try a revitalising hair treatment (see recipes on page 96)*
5 *Follow this with a warm shower and vigorously rub yourself with a sisal mitt and a rich moisturising soap, which will leave your skin deliciously clean and soft. If you have sensitive skin, use a sponge or a towelling mitt*
6 *Finish off with a quick cold shower*

Steam opens the pores and the perspiration engendered by the heat helps to flush out impurities.

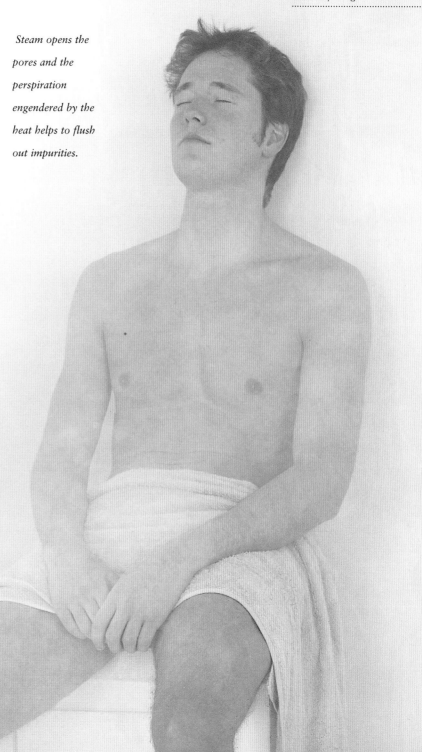

have any of the health conditions that preclude saunas, listed on page 27. Steam rooms are helpful, however, if your sinuses are blocked. The humidity of the steam aids decongestion. And unlike saunas, it is easy to recreate the therapeutic benefits of a steam treatment in your own bathroom. One way of doing it is to turn your entire bathroom into a steam room (see box above). This is a simple and effective means of bringing impurities to the surface and preparing your skin for a cleansing scrub that will leave it tingling and glowing with health.

Herbal detoxification

Lethargy, headaches, a bloated stomach and dull skin are all signs that your system is not working properly. The most frequent reason is that your body is overloaded with toxins. Detoxifying baths can help you to cleanse and revive your system.

Many factors can contribute to toxin build-up. Stress, for example, increases the quantity of chemicals such as cortisol, adrenalin and noradrenaline in your bloodstream. These chemicals slow down digestion, which leads to poor waste elimination. Excess amounts of caffeine, alcohol, nicotine and fatty and processed food are acid-forming, and a high level of acidity can eventually cause ill-health. The best antidote is to practise cleansing regimes, such as taking regular detoxifying baths.

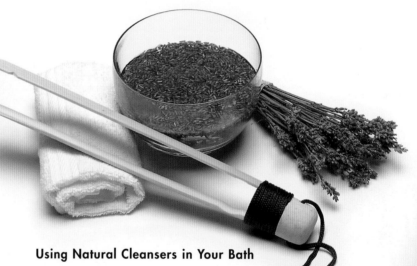

Herbal Facial Remedies

Bring a sparkle to your face by applying a herbal compress while you enjoy your reviving bath. Marsh mallow helps to purify the complexion and soothes dry skin. Clary sage heightens the libido and is good for oily skin. Lavender is kind to sensitive skin, and camomile is suitable for all skin types. Soak the compress in an infusion made from your chosen plant and place it on your face, keeping your eyes closed.

Using Natural Cleansers in Your Bath

Steep the herbs in hot water for 15–20 minutes. Strain and add the liquid to your bath. Tie the herbs in a cheesecloth or muslin sachet and attach to the tap, so that the sachet hangs under the running water. Apple cider vinegar has an energising and cleansing effect. Use about 2 cups. Nutmeg helps to increase perspiration. An infusion of root or powdered ginger speeds the metabolism. Use only small amounts. Add a blend of cedarwood, lavender and grapefruit essential oils; 1 drop of essential oil to 5ml (1 tsp) base oil.

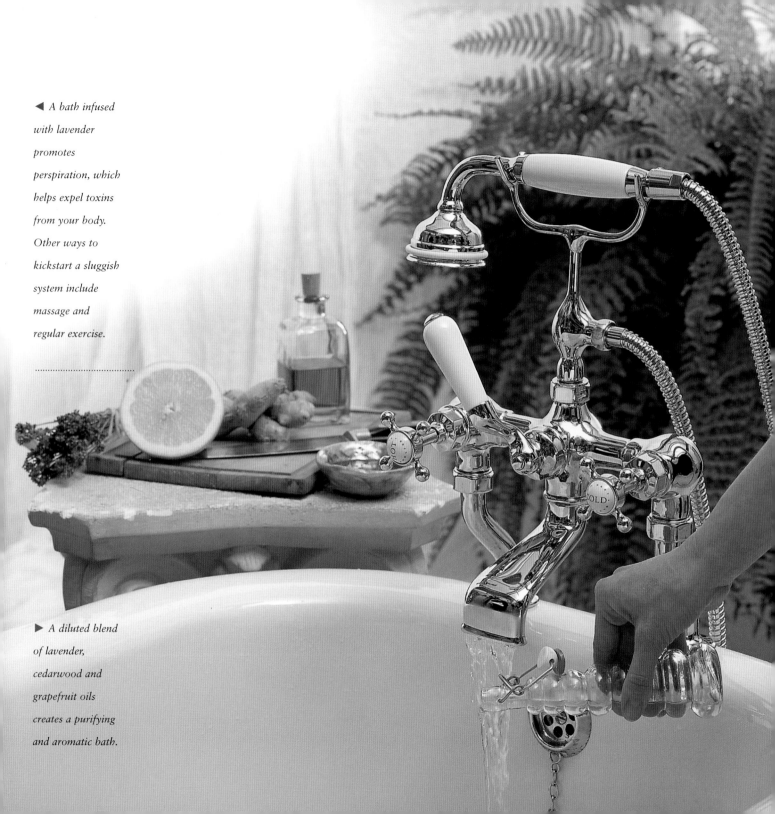

◀ *A bath infused with lavender promotes perspiration, which helps expel toxins from your body. Other ways to kickstart a sluggish system include massage and regular exercise.*

▶ *A diluted blend of lavender, cedarwood and grapefruit oils creates a purifying and aromatic bath.*

TURKISH BATHS

Bathing reached the height of sophistication during the Ottoman Empire (c.1300–1918). The Moors, like the Romans, delighted in water and steam, and built bathing houses, known as *hammams*, wherever they travelled.

The pillared halls, marble pools and fountains enhanced the delights of the Turkish hammam.

THE LIMITS OF THE MOORISH EMPIRE can be traced through the *hammams* that are dotted across Europe from Spain to Armenia — many of them still in use. Every town with a mosque had a bathhouse, usually fitted with marble pools and elaborately decorated with blue tiles, preferably from Izmir, assembled into stunning mosaics. Most *hammams* had separate sections or different days for men and women bathers. The baths that survive are as popular with locals and visitors to modern Turkey as they were in the great days of the sultans. The *hammam*

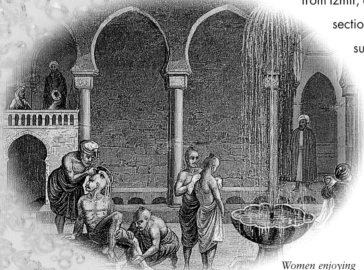

Women enjoying the benefits of a bathhouse in The Bath at Eroussa, *depicted by J.L. Gérôme (1870).*

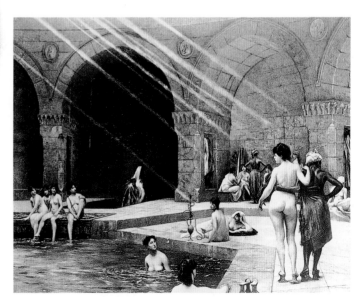

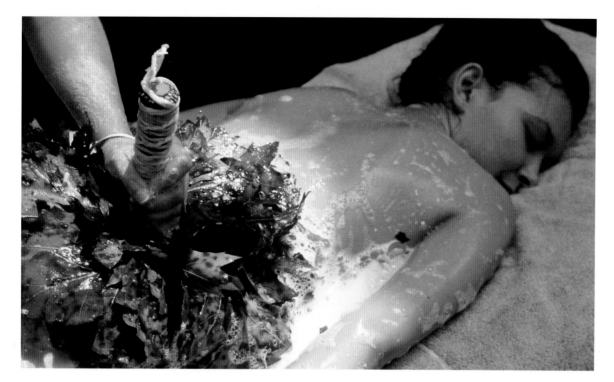

consisted of an inner steam room, surrounded by outer pools of hot and cold water. The inner room was an area set aside for contemplation and silence, while the outside pools were bustling places where sweets and refreshing drinks were served. Contacts were made here; the baths were a social place to network, discuss business or to exchange gossip. This social function was especially important for women, for whom bathing was the one reason they were allowed to leave their homes.

Roman Technology

The Moors benefited from the water technology of the Romans, using their aqueducts and their drainage systems to carry water to and from the town *hammams* and palaces. The 13th-century Alhambra Palace in Granada in southern Spain, world famous for its gardens and water features, has magnificent baths. They were the exclusive domain of the Moorish King of Granada and his harem of over 200 wives.

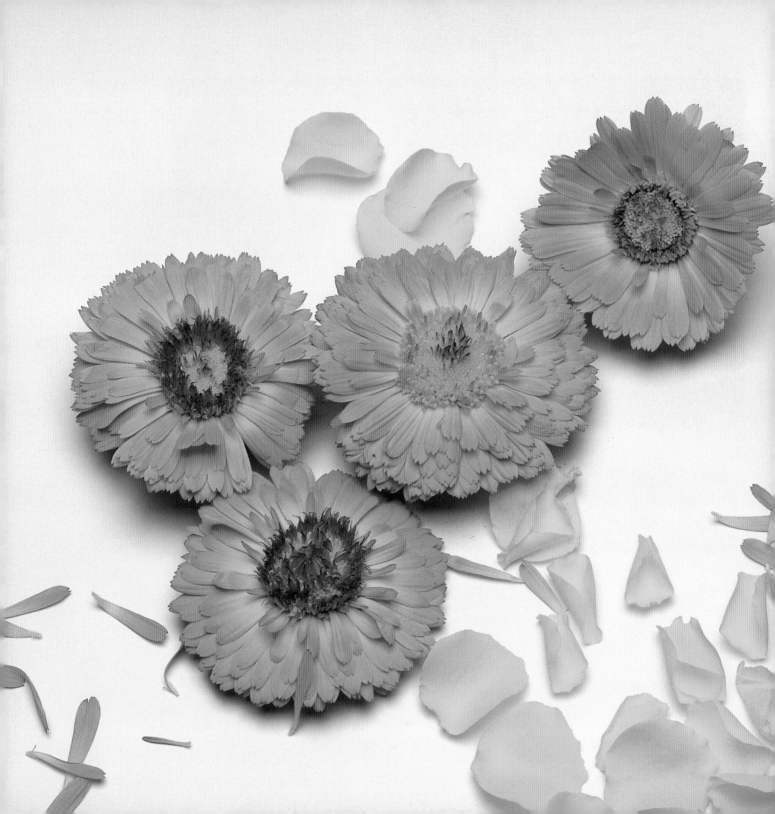

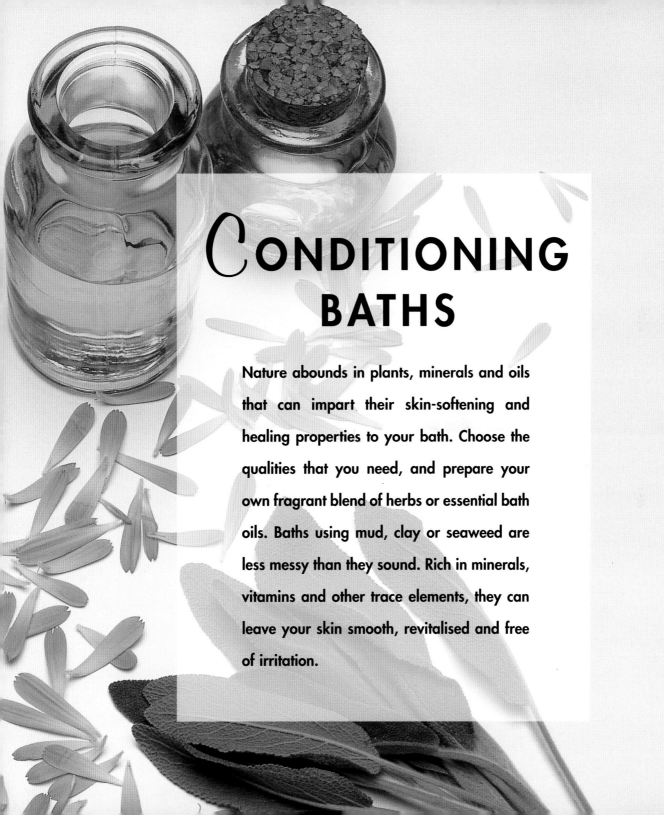

Conditioning Baths

Nature abounds in plants, minerals and oils that can impart their skin-softening and healing properties to your bath. Choose the qualities that you need, and prepare your own fragrant blend of herbs or essential bath oils. Baths using mud, clay or seaweed are less messy than they sound. Rich in minerals, vitamins and other trace elements, they can leave your skin smooth, revitalised and free of irritation.

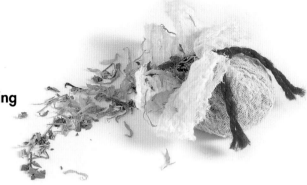

Moisturising baths

One of the simplest ways to counteract the drying effects of a long hot bath is by adding your favourite moisturising product to the water.

Unless you live in an area with very soft water, the chances are that regular bathing is dehydrating your skin. Applying moisturiser immediately after bathing is one solution. This can be time-consuming, however, or you may not want to apply moisturiser just before you get dressed, in case it leaves marks. An alternative is to put moisturiser into your bath, or to add natural moisturising ingredients, such as a handful of bran or oatmeal, so that you can cleanse and smooth your skin simultaneously. (You will need to sieve out the bran or oatmeal by placing a gauze cloth over the plug hole as the bath is drained.) Take a moisturising bath before bed, or if your skin is very dry, adopt the procedure morning and night. In this case, you will need a more convenient product.

Popular bath moisturisers sold in pharmacies and supermarkets can be effective, but tend to contain chemicals. It is better to choose natural ingredients, which work equally well.

Natural Oils

Adding a few drops of vegetable or plant oil is one of the easiest ways to create a moisturising bath. Do not use more than a couple of teaspoonfuls, or your bath will be too greasy. The warm water enables the oil to be absorbed more readily into your skin. When you emerge from your bath, there should be only the faintest residue of oil on your skin — and you will feel an immediate improvement in its texture.

- **For dry skin** choose avocado, sesame, wheat germ or castor oil. (Blend two of your favourites.)
- **For oily skin** choose lighter oils, such as camellia, calendula or safflower.
- **For normal skin** use almond, apricot, jojoba, or an oil rich in vitamin E.

Natural moisturisers rehydrate and soften. Tying fresh or dried camomile, lime blossom and elderflowers into a cheesecloth or muslin bag is a neat way to use them.

Facial Soaps

Even soaps that contain moisturisers can be too drying for your face. Products known as facial soaps tend to be soap-free and formulated from entirely different ingredients. They do not contain any harsh detergents and are designed to absorb grime from the skin's surface in a similar way to cleansing cream.

Natural Softeners

Softening herbs

Elderflowers, camomile and lime blossom all have a softening effect on the skin. Brew them into an infusion to add to your bath, or place a handful in a cheesecloth or muslin bag and allow the hot water to run through it.

Bran smoother

Regular bran or rice bran makes an excellent skin-smoother. Fill a cheesecloth or muslin sachet with the bran, and rub your skin with it while you are in the bath.

Oatmeal wash

Tie 250g (8oz) of dry rolled oats in a cheesecloth or muslin bag, and apply as an all-over skin softener. Or simmer the oats in water and, before they become too soft, strain the mixture through a sieve. Allow it to cool and add it to your bath water.

Oils should be used sparingly and only leave a slight sheen on the skin.

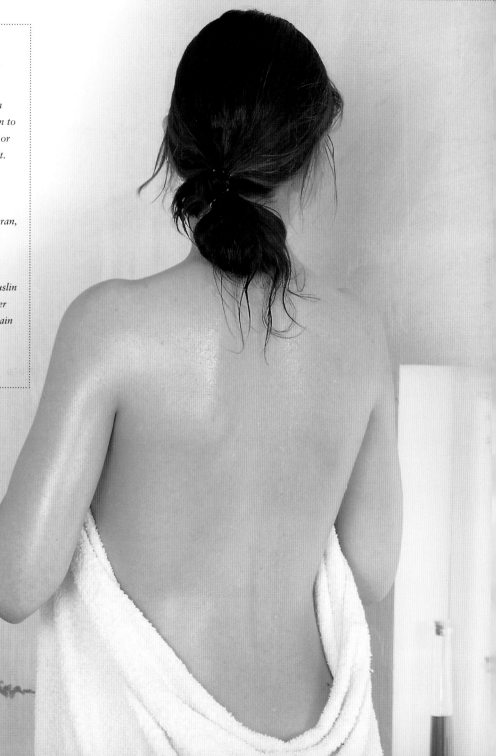

Essential oils

Few sensations can equal the bliss of sliding into a warm bath deliciously scented with a few drops of aromatic and health-giving essential oil.

The therapeutic effects of essential oils have been recognised for thousands of years, but the term aromatherapy dates from the 1920s. It was coined by the French cosmetic chemist René-Maurice Gattefosse, who carried out a lifetime's research into the properties of essential oils.

What are Essential Oils?

Essential oils encapsulate the distinctive fragrance of a plant and are present in tiny amounts in all aromatic flowers, leaves, seeds, grasses, roots and resins. They are complex chemical compounds, often comprising hundreds of separate substances, which determine their flavour and aroma and their particular therapeutic properties.

How to Use Essential Oils

Essential oils achieve their effects chiefly through inhalation and absorption through the skin from where they enter the bloodstream. A warm bath is one of the best methods of using them, because it enables you to absorb the oils simultaneously through your nose and skin.

Oils to Improve Your Skin

Regular use of essential oils can tone your skin and help to remedy problems. Mix your own conditioning bath oil from a combination of essential and carrier oils suitable for your skin type.

Skin type	Characteristics	Essential oils	Carrier oils
Normal	*Soft, supple and blemish-free*	*Geranium, rose, neroli, jasmine, lavender*	*Jojoba, sweet almond, olive, wheat germ, apricot kernel*
Dry	*Feels rough, taut and flaky*	*Camomile, jasmine, lemongrass, rose, sandalwood*	*Avocado, apricot kernel, sweet almond*
Oily	*Feels greasy to the touch*	*Cypress, orange, lemon, cedarwood, vetiver, lime*	*Grapeseed, sweet almond, apricot kernel*
Problem skin	*Prone to acne and spots*	*Grapefruit, lavender, tea-tree, juniper*	*Evening primrose, grapeseed*
Sensitive skin	*Prone to rashes, itches and redness*	*Camomile, rose, lavender*	*Grapeseed, evening primrose*
Mature skin	*Losing its elasticity; prone to sagging*	*Myrrh, rose, lavender, galbanum, frankincense, neroli, geranium*	*Evening primrose, jojoba, sweet almond, apricot kernel*

Never apply aromatherapy oils directly to the skin. Dilute them first in a carrier oil; apricot kernel, sweet almond, avocado, olive, safflower, sesame and wheat germ oils are just some to choose from. The essential oil should form 2–3 per cent of the solution. To prepare a massage oil, for example, blend one drop of essential oil with 5ml (1 tsp) of carrier oil. For a bath, you can either dilute 3–6 drops in a carrier oil or dissolve the drops of essential oil in the bath water.

Essential Advice

Always do a patch test before using any essential oil. Dilute in a carrier oil before applying to your skin. Essential oils last for 1–2 years — twice as long if kept chilled. Wrap them well or they will absorb other smells. Blended oils last for three months — so mix a limited amount as you need it. The exception is a mixture made with wheat germ oil (a natural preservative) which lasts for a year. An oil that is cloudy or smells more strongly than when you bought it is stale and should not be used. Essential oils are sensitive to light. Store them in dark glass bottles with stoppers, in a dark place. Do not keep oils in the bathroom — they will evaporate and become stale from the steam.

Aromatherapy oils, such as rosemary and rose oil, bring the distilled essence of a vast array of plants to your bathroom.

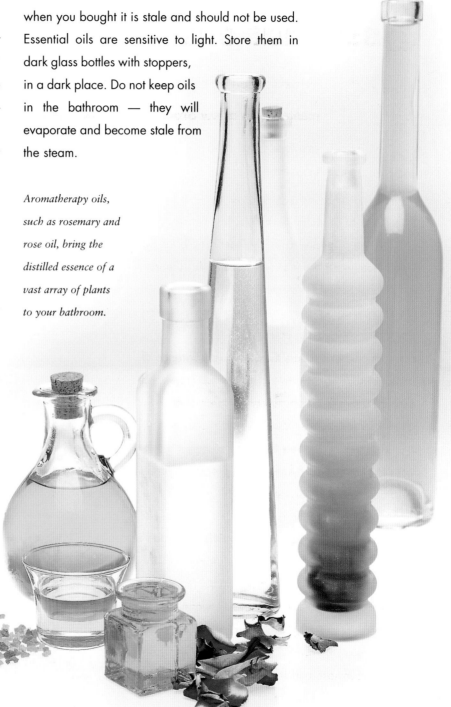

Smoothing and soothing salts

Mineral salts are essential to keep your skin in peak condition. Your body cannot make them, so you need to absorb them through your diet and through water — by drinking, but also by bathing. Water that is rich in minerals can work wonders.

In addition to keeping the skin healthy, mineral salts are vital to a range of bodily functions, including efficient blood circulation and the conduction of nerve impulses. The most important mineral salts are compounds of calcium, sodium, potassium and iron. Women are at greater risk of iron deficiency, because of menstruation. Calcium is crucial to all of us in keeping bones healthy and strong. As we get older, this element is more easily depleted.

Sea Salts

You may have noticed how a few days of bathing in the sea leaves your skin silky and blemish-free. This is because sea water is loaded with therapeutic minerals. Certain seas are renowned for their health-giving and skin-enhancing properties. The Dead Sea in Israel is claimed to be the richest source of mineral salts in the world. You can conjure up the resources of the Dead Sea in your own bath with salts bought over the counter from chemists or health food shops. They are packed with minerals, including bromides and sulphates of potassium, sodium, calcium and magnesium. These are easily absorbed by the skin and, in addition to improving its texture, they can help to alleviate conditions such as psoriasis and eczema. Mineral salt baths also ease aches and pains.

Epsom Salts

Epsom salts are another readily available and rich source of minerals. A bath in Epsom salts increases perspiration, helps flush out toxins, soothes aching muscles and leaves your skin refreshed and smooth. Add a few drops of lavender essential oil, diluted in carrier oil (see Essential oils, pages 38–9) to boost skin-conditioning properties.

Mineral salts used in combination with lavender essential oil can smooth skin and soothe soreness.

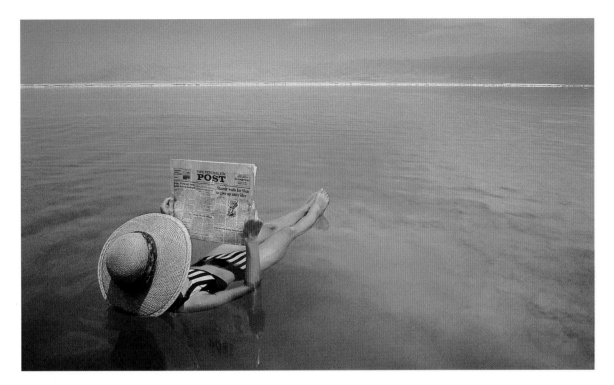

The Dead Sea in Israel is packed with healing mineral salts that can banish blemishes, enhance skin texture and relieve severe skin problems. Dead Sea salts can be obtained over the counter for home use.

Caution Epsom salts are potent and must be used with care. Do not stay in the bath longer than 20 minutes. Bathing longer does not increase the benefits and can make you feel weak. Be especially cautious if you have hypertension, diabetes, or a heart condition. If in any doubt seek your doctor's advice about the temperature and individual conditions that are safe for you.

Stimulating and Simple

Salt baths stimulate the skin and promote the removal of toxins. They boost blood circulation and their absorption helps major organs, such as the liver and the kidneys, to function more efficiently. The by-product of these benefits to your system is smooth, flawless skin. And mineral salts are practical — they dissolve into the water without leaving a residue.

A Therapeutic Bath

The ideal temperature for a therapeutic mineral salt bath is 30–37°C (86–98.5°F). A temperature of 25–28°C (77–82.5°F) provides a more stimulating effect. Add about 1.8kg (4lb) of salt to the water. Lie in the bath for 10–20 minutes.

Glorious mud

A mud or clay treatment may sound messy — but professional products can make it easy. The substances used, dug from deep within the earth, come in an array of colours, and are rich in minerals that smooth the skin and soothe aching limbs.

Mud and clay treatments have been used throughout history and continue to be a staple therapy of most health spas. They improve skin texture and draw out impurities. Mud and clay can also alleviate painful conditions such as rheumatism and arthritis. The substances used are extracted from deep down in the earth in areas where minerals are plentiful.

Muds and clays can be red, green, yellow, white, black, brown, even pink — depending on their place of origin. There are famous sources in Morocco, Italy, the Black Sea and the Dead Sea. They are suitable for all skin types but are especially beneficial for oily and problem skins. White clay is best for oily skins because it is naturally astringent. If your skin is dry choose one of the softer, brown clays or muds. Green clay is especially good for acne and Dead Sea mud for other skin problems.

During certain mud treatments carried out at a spa — where you lie in huge quantities of mud, for example — it is customary to leave the left arm and heart area mud-free, to avoid over-stimulating the system.

Mud Facial

The mud pack is probably the oldest and most effective face mask. It cleanses, soothes, tones and makes you feel wonderfully refreshed. Choose a mud product recommended for your skin type.

Home Mud Bath

Most health food shops and some chemists sell conveniently packaged mud or clay products. With a little planning, you can enjoy a mud bath in your own bathroom (see page 93).

Caution Do not try a mud bath treatment if you have any of the following conditions: heart disease, hypertension, diabetes, epilepsy.

When you have a complete body mud wrap at a spa you will be wrapped in a foil sheet to retain the heat generated from the mud and by your body. This helps to make the mud work more efficiently.

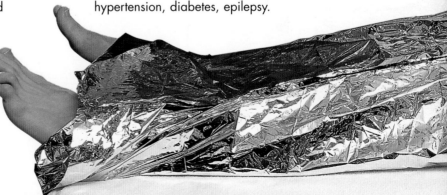

To Make a Mud Pack

You Will Need

180g (6oz) Fuller's earth powder, 1 cup (250ml/8fl oz) lemon or lime juice, 10ml (2 tsp) almond oil, 5ml (1 tsp) clear honey, 1 drop sandalwood essential oil

1 *For maximum benefit, exfoliate first.*
2 *Mix the mud or Fuller's earth into a thick paste with the lemon or lime juice. Add enough warm water to warm and liquefy the mixture.*
3 *Stir in the almond oil, honey and sandalwood oil and blend well.*
4 *Spread the mixture over your entire body, starting with your feet. Ask a partner to do the parts of your back and middle shoulders that you cannot reach. If this is not possible, just focus on specific areas; thighs, to boost circulation and treat cellulite; arms, legs, or back for problem skin.*
5 *Cover the coated areas in plastic wrap or foil to retain the heat generated by the mud or clay.*
6 *Leave on for 15–20 minutes, then shower off under tepid water. Follow with a warm bath infused with a few drops of almond oil.*
7 *Drink plenty of water afterwards to rehydrate.*

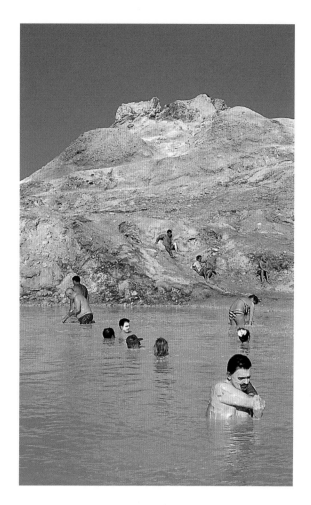

Sources of therapeutic muds and clays which may be present in thermal springs, like this one on Vulcano Island, off northern Sicily, have been prized for centuries by those seeking pain relief and skin health.

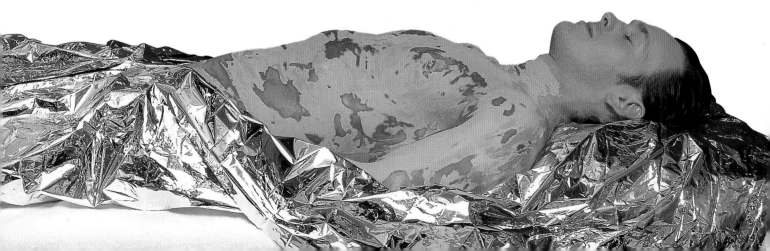

Seaweed baths

Smoother skin, increased vitality, even inch-loss on targeted areas of your body: discover the amazing benefits of thalassotherapy (the practice of using seaweed and sea water to treat a variety of health conditions).

Seaweed is the generic term for over 20,000 species of sea plants and algae (single-celled organisms) that inhabit the world's oceans and seas. It is packed with vitamins, minerals and other beneficial elements that help to soothe, detoxify, heal skin, boost immunity and lower blood pressure. It may even induce temporary weight loss.

How to Use Seaweed

The simplest ways to experience the benefits of seaweed are through wraps and baths (see page 92). You can buy fresh seaweed from major health food shops and Japanese delicatessens — always choose organic — but it is easier to opt for the ready-to-use dried powders and bath sachets. Seaweed

Give Yourself a Seaweed Wrap

You Will Need

180g (6oz) concentrated dried micronised seaweed powder (available from health food shops and some Japanese shops)
2 tbsp (30ml/1fl oz) carrier oil (eg almond)
2 drops lavender and/or rosemary essential oil (see pages 100–103)
1 *For maximum effect, prepare your skin by exfoliating and taking a warm shower or bath.*

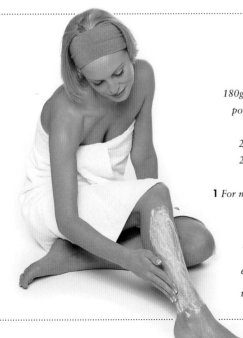

◀ *Before applying a wrap, exfoliate all over, wash in warm water and dry gently.*

2 *Mix the dried seaweed powder with a little warm water (enough to warm it and make it more fluid).*
3 *Blend the carrier oil with the essential oil(s) and add to the seaweed mixture to make a thick paste.*
4 *Apply the paste over your entire body, starting with the feet. Ask someone to help you cover the parts you cannot reach such as your back.*
5 *To hold in the heat generated by the wrap, cover yourself in plastic wrap or foil.*
6 *Keep on for 20–30 minutes.*
7 *Rinse off under a warm shower. Remember to drink plenty of water afterwards.*

treatments are detoxifying, so always make sure you drink plenty of spring water afterwards to continue the process and to rehydrate your body.

Thalassotherapy Treatments

Thalassotherapy, which takes its name from the Greek word for sea, is now available at most health farms, salons and spas. Treatments include seaweed wraps, marine algae baths and sea-water sprays and showers. Seaweed is filled with vitamins, minerals, natural trace elements, amino acids and enzymes — including large amounts of vitamin C, along with iodine, gamma linoleic acid, beta carotene, chlorophyll, kelp, calcium, mag-nesium, potassium, phosphorus and sodium — all of which are easily absorbed into the skin. It stimulates circulation, soothes muscular aches and pains and reduces cholesterol. It can also be useful as part of a shape-control programme. This is because regular seaweed treatments lead to more efficient elimination of toxins and can also stimulate the metabolism to function more effectively. Combined with a healthy diet and plenty of exercise, a thalassotherapy regime can work wonders in toning the body.

Seaweed has also been shown to kill bacteria. It can heal and soothe skin conditions such as eczema and psoriasis, and is beneficial in clearing problem skin.

Powdered seaweed can be mixed to a paste with water and essential oil to make a seaweed wrap.

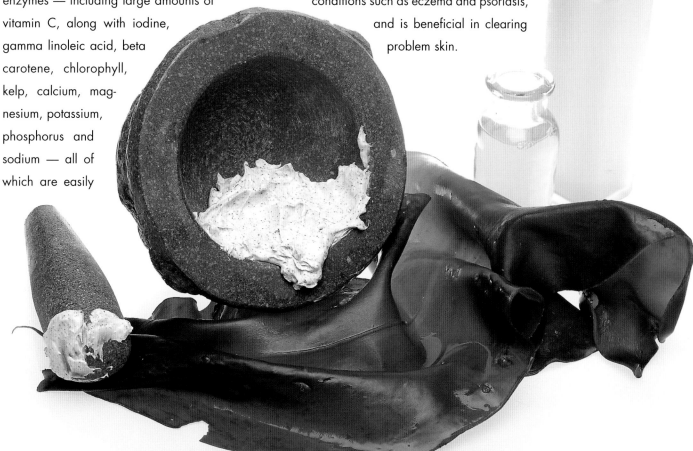

HEALING SPRINGS

The most luxurious way to indulge in the rejuvenating effects of mineral-rich natural waters is to visit a spa that offers mineral water therapies. Here you can relax in a mineral bath or swim in a mineral pool.

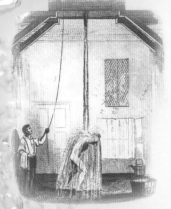

Taking a shower in mineral water at Malvern spa in the hills of Western England, in 1835.

THE HEALING POWERS OF mineral waters have been renowned for centuries. The ancient Greeks and Romans knew the therapeutic qualities of waters enriched with minerals such as calcium, potassium, sulphur and magnesium. They recognised that bathing in certain waters alleviated a variety of ailments.

Following the decline of the Roman Empire, the health benefits of mineral waters were largely neglected. It was not until the 18th century that Roman baths were revived, and new 'watering holes' became fashionable. The legacy of that period can be seen in spas around the world to which people travel in search of relief from conditions ranging from skin disorders to rheumatism and arthritis.

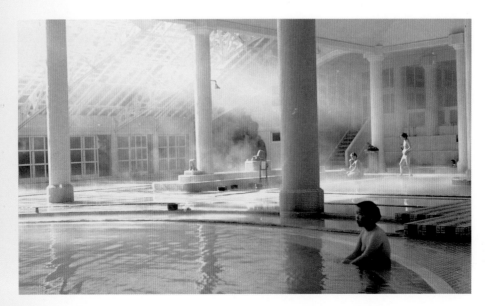

Steam baths on Japan's northern island of Hokkaido, where the hot springs of Noboribetsu provide 100,000 gallons of hot water a day.

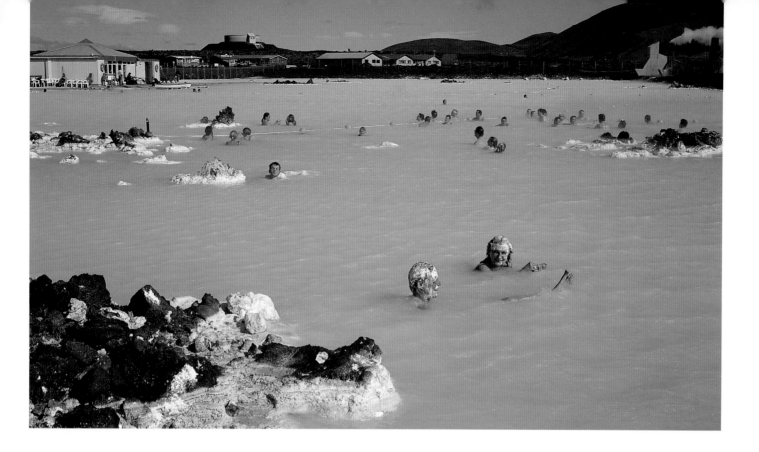

The Secrets of the Spa

The composition of spa water varies according to the region where it occurs. Some waters are rich in iron; others are known for their calcium or sulphur content. Spa water has a variety of therapeutic effects, depending on the mineral it contains (see pages 104–5). Saturnia, a spa in central Italy, is rich in sulphur which is beneficial for skin and muscular disorders. Many spas today, particularly in Europe, specialise in medically supervised treatments for conditions such as rheumatism, arthritis and eczema.

Some kinds of spa water are better taken internally, as a drink, but the majority are recommended for both drinking and bathing. At some spas, such as those in Iceland and the United States, thermal waters bubble up from naturally occurring hot springs — all you need do is hop in and enjoy the warming, therapeutic effects of the warm water amid snow and ice. Native North Americans were using the healing powers of hot springs long before the arrival of the Europeans, and knew of countless such sources, including the famous Saratoga Springs in New York, kept secret by the Iroquois until 1767.

The Blue Lagoon, near Grindavik in Iceland, where people can enjoy swimming in warm therapeutic water. Iceland possesses more than 100 hot springs, or geysers, of volcanic origin that produce boiling water instead of lava.

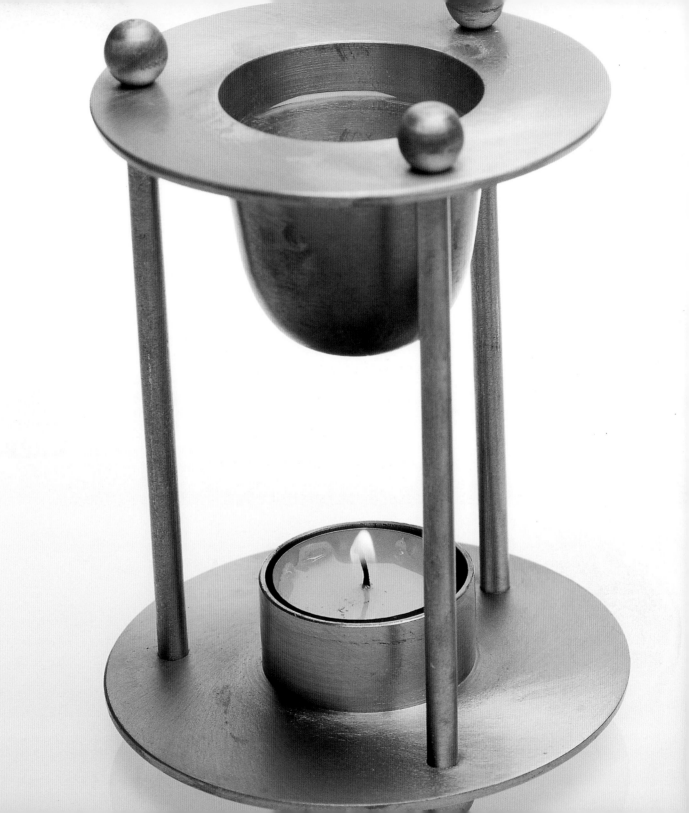

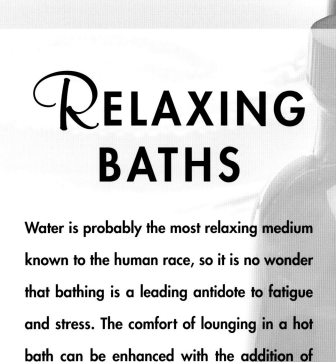

RELAXING BATHS

Water is probably the most relaxing medium known to the human race, so it is no wonder that bathing is a leading antidote to fatigue and stress. The comfort of lounging in a hot bath can be enhanced with the addition of natural ingredients that promote relaxation or lull your body ready for sleep. The bath is the perfect place for a gentle massage. Bathing can be made even more sensual with the help of mood-enhancing ingredients.

Flowers and foods

Fruity, flowery bath preparations not only smell wonderful in the water, they also have an instant feel-good effect on the psyche and many therapeutic benefits for the skin.

Commercial preparations may smell good, but they are almost always synthetically produced. To experience the full, natural qualities, use the real thing. Add fruit, flowers or food directly to the bath, or apply them in the form of packs and tonics. Fruits, flowers and food essences can make a delicious and therapeutic addition to your bathtime ritual. They can relieve stress and enhance the texture and appearance of your skin.

Imagine for a moment the scent of fresh limes. Even thinking about their specific citrus aroma can be refreshing. It is no surprise, then, that they are among the fragrances that can give you an energy boost, offering instant relief from fatigue.

Fruit and Other Foods

Milk for silky, smooth, soft skin. Not just a favourite with Cleopatra — Indian women have used milk for centuries. Pour as much powdered or fresh milk as you wish into a hot bath.

Grapes for blemish-free skin. Add grape juice to your bath, or make a decoction of vine leaves for a cleansing, antiseptic effect.

Ginger helps stimulate circulation. It is warming and aromatic. Add a few tablespoonfuls of ground ginger, or a decoction made from the fresh root.

Pineapple contains a natural enzyme that helps to improve the skin. Add freshly squeezed pineapple juice to the bath, or use it on your face as a toner.

Honey has natural healing, antiseptic qualities. It helps blemished skin and is very moisturising. Stir a few tablespoonfuls into your bath.

Citrus fruits (lemons, oranges, limes) smooth the texture of the skin. Grate the rind and add it to the bath. Apply lemon juice directly to elbows, feet and knees. Or place the rinds in a cheesecloth or muslin bag and rub the skin briskly to exfoliate.

Tropical fruits (melons, papaya, cantaloupe) possess skin-beautifying properties. Papaya, especially, is rich in enzymes that can improve skin texture. Mash these fruits into a pulp and apply them to the face or body. Leave for about 15 minutes and rinse off. Or add some ground almond meal to the fruits and use the mixture to exfoliate your skin while you bath.

Cornmeal and oatmeal are good exfoliants — oatmeal is beneficial to dry, irritated skin. Add them

A wide array of fruits, flowers, spices, cereal grains and other natural substances are good for the condition of your skin — applied directly, mashed to a paste, or added to the bath.

directly to the bath, or make them into a paste with some hot water and a tablespoonful of lemon juice. Massage over body. Rinse off.

Strawberries soothe skin irritations and sensitive skin. Mash them up, apply them to the skin as a pack and rinse off.

Peach is helpful for inflamed, blotchy skin. Mash the fruit and make into a pack. Apply to the face or body for 15 minutes. Rinse off.

Vanilla smells warm and comforting. Add a few drops of vanilla essence to your bath.

Flowers

Honeysuckle calms skin irritations. Make an infusion from the blossom, and add to the bath.

Iris helps improve circulation and has a calming effect. Scatter petals in your bathwater.

Marigold helps dry, sensitive skin. Add an infusion of the flowers to your bath.

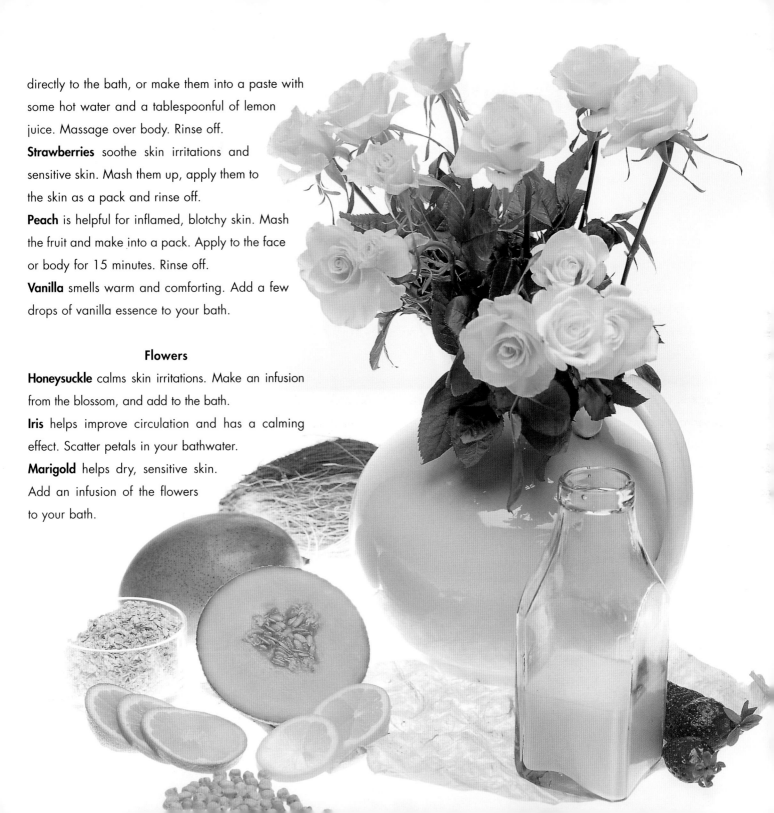

Essential oils for relaxation

The distilled scents of plants can have a powerful effect on mind and body.

For instant relaxation, discover the calming aromas of essential oils.

Imagine your favorite scent. Think about how it feels to inhale its particular aroma. Whether you realise it or not, your choice of fragrance — be it from scent, soap, or freshly cut flowers — is determined by the way it makes you feel. The knowledge that smells affect the psyche is not new; the mood-altering properties of various aromas have all been recognised for centuries and the perfume industry thrives on our emotive response to fragrance.

The most powerfully therapeutic scents are those that emanate from essential oils (see pages 38–9).

Recommended Blends

General Relaxation Formula
5 drops neroli • 5 drops lavender • 5 drops lemon*

For Anxiety
5 drops lavender • 5 drops geranium • 5 drops rose*

Calming Formula
5 drops clary sage • 5 drops lavender •
5 drops lemon*

* diluted with carrier oil

'Essential' Face Tips
The nearer an essential oil is to your nose, the more rapid the effect on your psyche. Apply a few drops, diluted in a carrier oil, to a face flannel and place it across your nose and cheeks while you relax in the bath. Meanwhile soothe your eyes and tone the delicate eye area with pads soaked in an infusion of cornflower petals (45g/1½oz to 500ml/2 cups).

In aromatherapy, essential oils are selected for their uplifting, calming, or even aphrodisiac qualities. The smell of each oil triggers a specific effect. Drawn from the core of nature itself, the oils possess healing properties not found in any of their synthetic counterparts. When you smell an essential oil, the molecules quickly pass into the bloodstream, which disperses them throughout your system. In addition to affecting specific organs, essential oils act upon the limbic part of the brain (its most primitive area, which is concerned with emotions). The mental and emotional influence is determined by the oil you choose. Some, such as camomile, work on areas of the brain and nervous system to induce a deep state of relaxation and inner calm.

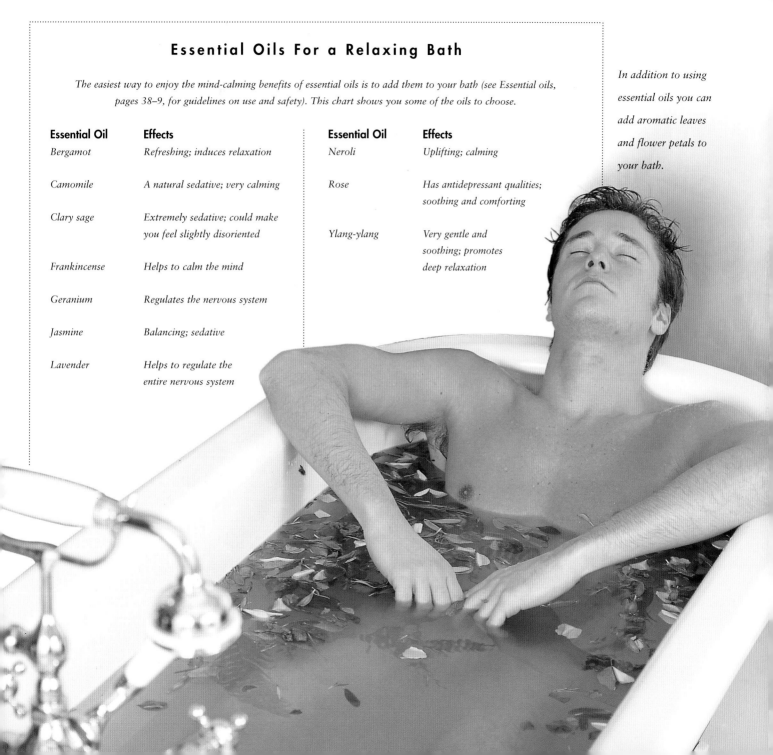

Essential Oils For a Relaxing Bath

The easiest way to enjoy the mind-calming benefits of essential oils is to add them to your bath (see Essential oils, pages 38–9, for guidelines on use and safety). This chart shows you some of the oils to choose.

In addition to using essential oils you can add aromatic leaves and flower petals to your bath.

Essential Oil	Effects	Essential Oil	Effects
Bergamot	Refreshing; induces relaxation	Neroli	Uplifting; calming
Camomile	A natural sedative; very calming	Rose	Has antidepressant qualities; soothing and comforting
Clary sage	Extremely sedative; could make you feel slightly disoriented	Ylang-ylang	Very gentle and soothing; promotes deep relaxation
Frankincense	Helps to calm the mind		
Geranium	Regulates the nervous system		
Jasmine	Balancing; sedative		
Lavender	Helps to regulate the entire nervous system		

$\mathscr{A}$ handful of herbs

Feeling stressed? In need of some tender loving care? A relaxing hot bath steeped with soothing herbs can relieve tension, calm discomfort and bring feelings of serenity.

Herbal remedies have existed for centuries. They are a foundation stone of modern medicine, yet few people feel knowledgeable about their uses, and many easy home treatments have been forgotten.

There are differing approaches to herbalism. The Eastern (Chinese and Ayurvedic) method is based mainly on the ability of herbs to 'rebalance the energies' throughout the body. The Western perspective concentrates on their 'active' ingredients. Herbs can be as potent as laboratory-made drugs, many of which were derived from plants. Aspirin, for example, originated from the

Herb Chart

Choose from the herbs in this chart, and use in one of the following ways. Steep the herbs in hot water, cool slightly and add to the bath. Or wrap them in a cheesecloth or muslin bag and hang it from the tap, so that the hot water runs through it.

Herb	When to use	How to use
Camomile	*Use when feeling restless, anxious, to calm a 'nervous' stomach due to stress, or to help stomach cramps.*	*Make a tea from camomile teabags. Empty the solution into the bathwater.*
Lavender	*Has a balancing effect on the nervous system. Helps calm the mind and leaves you feeling more peaceful.*	*Use dried flowers alone or in combination with camomile.*
Lime flowers	*Their scent has a gentle, soothing effect that assists mental relaxation.*	*Infuse and add to the bathwater.*
Lemon balm	*Helps you to loosen up and unwind generally.*	*Only useful when fresh — otherwise the action is negligible.*
Passion flower	*A natural sedative, it helps you to feel more serene.*	*Add the leaves or the flowers to your bath.*

white willow; digitalis, a medication used for heart disease, came from the foxglove. There is said to be a herb for every human ailment.

Herbs contain complex substances, including essential vitamins, minerals and oils. These ingredients are assimilated by the body, either internally or through the application of poultices and compresses, and bathing in herb-infused water.

In the Bath

Adding herbs to your bath is a gentler, less concentrated way of using herbs than eating or drinking them, but can be equally therapeutic. When you add herbs to your bath, they have a twofold effect. They are absorbed by your skin — carrying their active ingredients — but you acquire added benefit from breathing in their calming vapours. The effect is similar to that of adding essential oils to your bath.

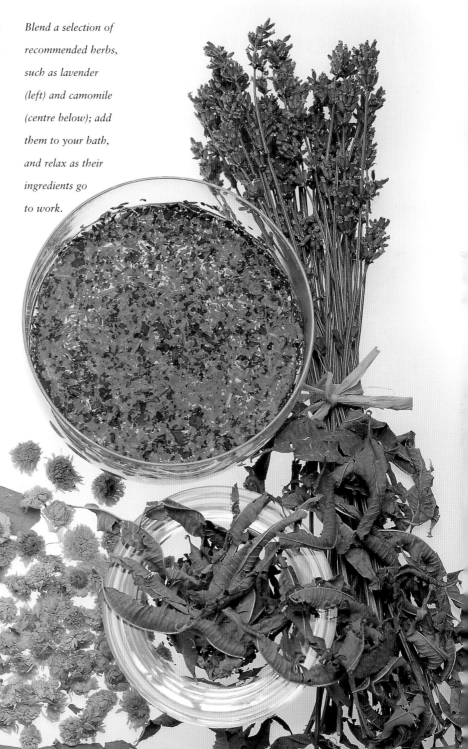

Blend a selection of recommended herbs, such as lavender (left) and camomile (centre below); add them to your bath, and relax as their ingredients go to work.

Sensual baths

Transform your bathroom into a haven of pleasure and relaxation, where you can indulge your senses and recharge both physically and mentally.

Genuine relaxation should leave you feeling refreshed and energised. It's an opportunity to calm both body and mind. And sometimes the simplest methods have the most profound effect. Don't think of your bathroom as just a place to wash in. It can double as your personal sanctuary.

Sensual Pleasures

Try to surround yourself with objects that are not merely functional but also pleasing to the senses. Beautiful bottles, scented soaps, sea sponges, plants and unusual containers for basic items enhance the most ordinary bathroom. To tone down harsh

How Chakras Work

Chakras are energy centres located at key points in the body from the base to the top of the spine. They can be stimulated by massage and the energy emitted by colours and light.

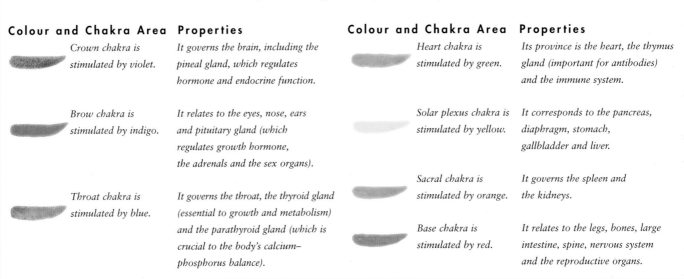

Colour and Chakra Area

	Colour and Chakra Area	**Properties**
	Crown chakra is stimulated by violet.	*It governs the brain, including the pineal gland, which regulates hormone and endocrine function.*
	Brow chakra is stimulated by indigo.	*It relates to the eyes, nose, ears and pituitary gland (which regulates growth hormone, the adrenals and the sex organs).*
	Throat chakra is stimulated by blue.	*It governs the throat, the thyroid gland (essential to growth and metabolism) and the parathyroid gland (which is crucial to the body's calcium–phosphorus balance).*

Colour and Chakra Area **Properties**

	Colour and Chakra Area	**Properties**
	Heart chakra is stimulated by green.	*Its province is the heart, the thymus gland (important for antibodies) and the immune system.*
	Solar plexus chakra is stimulated by yellow.	*It corresponds to the pancreas, diaphragm, stomach, gallbladder and liver.*
	Sacral chakra is stimulated by orange.	*It governs the spleen and the kidneys.*
	Base chakra is stimulated by red.	*It relates to the legs, bones, large intestine, spine, nervous system and the reproductive organs.*

lighting install a rheostat dimmer and add a few candles. The warm glow of candlelight has a calming effect. Burning your favourite scented candles or essential oil can also enhance a sensual setting. Scents for a sensual mood include rose, jasmine, ylang-ylang, patchouli, frankincense, sandalwood, neroli and geranium.

Caution Take care never to leave aromatherapy burners or candles unattended. Always extinguish them after taking your bath.

Colour Therapy

The colours in your surroundings have a powerful effect. Colour is energy; it results from wavelengths of 'visible light', which vibrate at different speeds. Colour has long been recognised as a valuable healing aid. As early as 1550 BC, the ancient Egyptians compiled a list of colour cures. They believed that the energy of each colour affected different processes in the body. This view is shared by traditional Indian medicine, which holds that the body contains seven major energy centres, known as chakras. Each chakra governs specific organs and glands and is stimulated by a different colour of light.

Transform your bathroom into a luxurious space and indulge your senses. Light candles, burn aromatic oils and have plenty of soft bath towels to complete the calming experience.

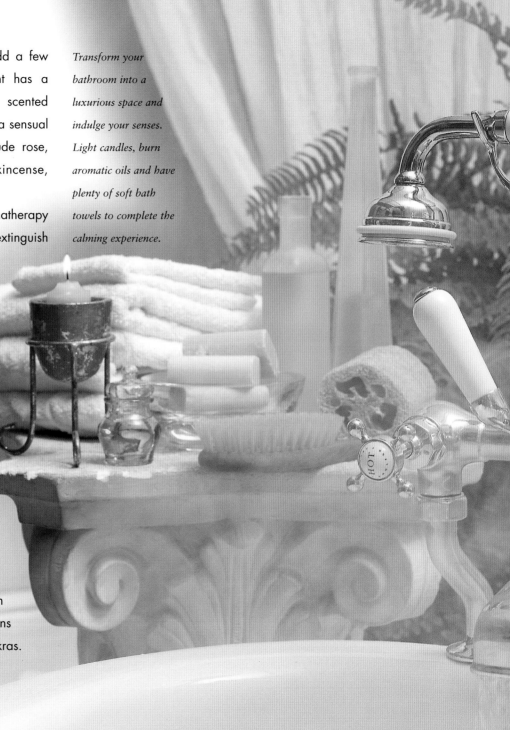

Massage

You don't have to be an expert to give yourself a massage. The simplest pressure can bring benefits to the skin and underlying soft tissue — such as muscles, ligaments and tendons — and engender feelings of relaxation throughout your body and mind.

Massage is a virtually instinctive response to pain. Think of how you rub a sore muscle or knead an aching shoulder. Even the most elementary massage helps to stimulate the circulation, dilate blood vessels and relax muscular tension. It's not surprising, therefore, that massage techniques have evolved worldwide throughout human history.

Western Massage

The best known Western method is the Swedish massage, which is based on long, sweeping strokes all over the body. Lymphatic drainage is also very popular in health and beauty salons. It consists of a deep tissue massage aimed at dispersing toxins along the lymphatic path, which contribute to conditions such as bloatedness and cellulite.

Eastern Massage

Eastern techniques, such as Shiatsu, Thai massage, or Chinese acupressure, apply pressure to key points along the meridians, or channels, that are believed to carry energy through the body. They aim to release blocked energy and restore the balanced flow on which good health depends.

Self-massage

Everyone can benefit from self-massage. And the bath is a good place to practise, because your muscles are warm and receptive from the heat of the water. Try the techniques described here. Massage with your hands or a sisal mitt, lubricated with your favourite creamy soap, oil or bath gel. Always massage towards your heart.

Water Massage

A popular health spa treatment is to lie in a bath equipped with rotating water jets that massage your body. Alternatively, you can have yourself massaged with a hoselike attachment that applies a jet of water to pressure points around your body. Recreate this effect in the bath, using a shower hose. Direct the water all over your body in circular motions, in the same way as if you were massaging with your hands.

Massage Strokes

Try these strokes, beginning with effleurage ("gentle touching"), to discover the delights of massage. By massaging the neck, shoulders, arms, legs, and feet you will rapidly learn to detect and soothe areas of muscle tightness.

Apply a fragrant oil, warmed in the palms of your hands, to make your massage more relaxing.

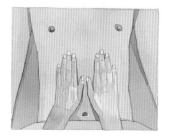

Effleurage
Press lightly in long continuous, skimming motions all over the body. This is especially useful to ease congestion in the stomach area. Keep the fingers close together with fingertips slightly raised.

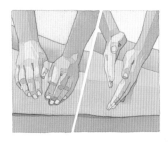

Tapotement
Apply a combination of cupping and chopping movements quickly all over the skin. This tones circulation, especially along the hips, the backs of the thighs, and the calves.

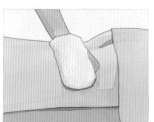

Friction massage
Rub speedily backward and forward with a friction mitt or hemp glove to stimulate blood flow.

Pressure points
Press key points on the body, using the fingers or thumb (see body massage diagram on page 21).

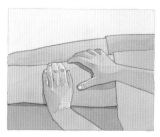

Petrissage
"Knead" the muscles in a circular direction, using the palm of the hand and the balls of the fingers, trapping rather than stroking the skin. This helps to relax stiff muscles.

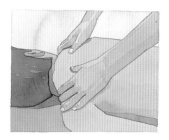

Deeper muscle massage
Use your fingers and thumb to "rotate" the muscles in small upward circular movements. This is especially soothing on the upper arms and shoulders.

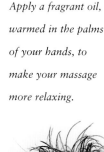
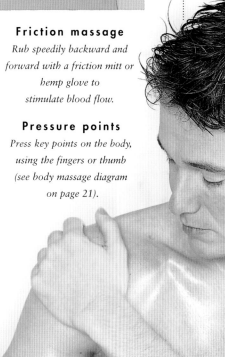

Baths to help you sleep

You can cope with the occasional sleepless night, but what do you do when you continuously find yourself tossing and turning in the small hours of the morning?

If external distractions are preventing you from falling asleep, the solutions are fairly easy. Invest in a pair of earplugs. Keep your bedroom as dark as possible with curtains or blinds. Check also that your bedroom is neither too hot nor too cold; for a good night's sleep, it should be between 18° and 21°C (64° and 70°F). To prevent an overburdened stomach from keeping you awake, avoid eating after 6 pm, apart perhaps from a herbal tea. And if all these tactics continue to leave you alert at 3 o'clock in the morning, try the simplest remedy of all; a sleep-inducing bath just before bed.

Relaxing Baths

It sounds too easy to be effective. Yet lacing your bath with soporific ingredients can ensure you have a restful night and you awake feeling refreshed.

Lavender and camomile Both of these plants can help you relax before you go to bed. Dilute 5–8 drops of essential oil of lavender or camomile in a carrier oil (see Essential oils, pages 38–9), and add it to your bath. Or make an infusion with lavender and camomile flowers (see A handful of herbs, pages 54–5). Save some of the oil blend and rub a little on the soles of your feet before getting into bed for an even more potent effect. Enhance the benefits by sipping a cup of herbal tea after your bath.

Hops can also have a tranquillising effect. Make an infusion to add to the bath by steeping a handful of the flowers in hot water, or tie the flowers in a sachet and attach them to the tap.

Skullcap is a medicinal, somewhat bitter herb, which belongs to the mint family. It won't smell great in the bath, but is worth trying because it can be remarkably effective. Skullcap acts on the nervous system to promote a feeling of deep relaxation.

Valerian This is renowned for its calming, sleep-inducing properties. Use it sparingly (see safety note right). Valerian acts like a tranquilliser, thanks largely

A warm bath infused with sedative herbs can lull your body and mind into a state of readiness for a night of peaceful slumber.

to one of its volatile oils, isovaleric acid. Its soporific effects are balanced by a number of other ingredients that make up its complex chemical structure, so that unlike conventional sedative drugs, it does not leave the system feeling sluggish and slow. The best way to use it is to make an infusion, using fresh valerian, which you add to your bath. Other herbs that combat sleeplessness include **Passion flower** and **lemon balm** (see A handful of herbs, pages 54–5). They can be used on their own or combined with any of the herbs mentioned above. **Caution** It is dangerous to fall asleep in the bath. When you begin to feel drowsy, get out of the bath immediately.

Experiment to find the tranquillising herb, or combination of herbs, that relaxes you best. Steep the fresh herb in the bathwater, make an infusion of fresh or dried herbs, or hang a generously bulging sachet under the running tap.

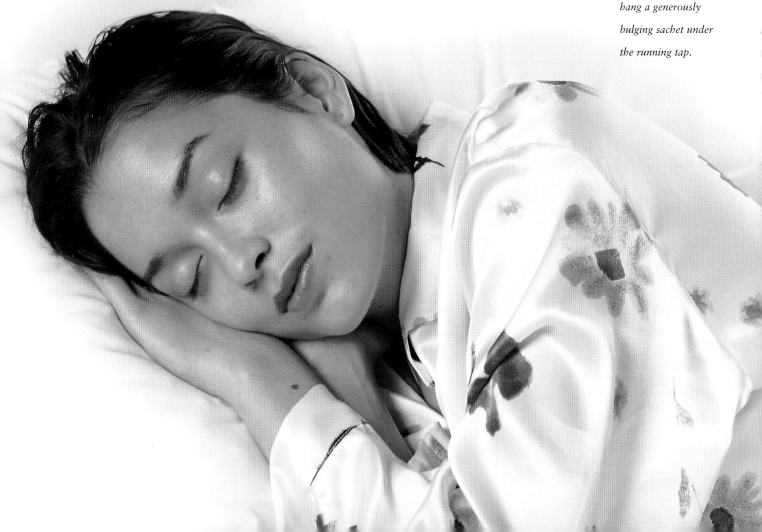

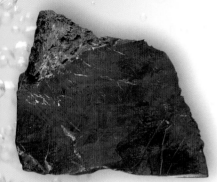

WATER ELIXIRS

The idea of transforming water into an elixir charged with healing energies was known to the ancient Egyptians and the early native North Americans.

Gemstones such as jasper (which can be vibrant red or calm green) are said to emit healing energy.

WATER ELIXIRS ARE BASED on the concept that pure spring water can be charged with the healing energy of crystals, colours and plants. This is said to be because water is capable of 'memorising' the specific energetic vibration that is the sign of a natural healing substance. Today water elixirs are prescribed by therapists, although it is illegal in some countries to claim they have medicinal value.

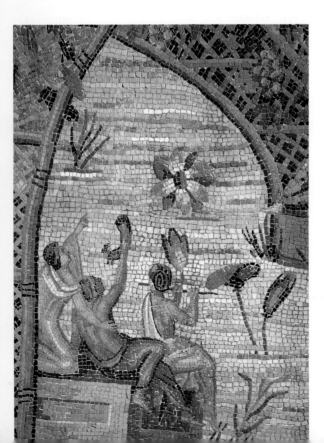

Roman women of the 1st–2nd century AD on the banks of the River Nile. The Romans believed in the mystical powers of water, crystals and colours.

Celestial Icicles

Crystals have always been a source of fascination. In ancient times they were thought to be made from the frozen water of the heavens; the word crystal is derived from the Greek for ice. These celestial icicles were believed to be steeped in mystical properties. The Chinese of 5,000 years ago used jade to strengthen and heal the body. European knights of the Middle Ages wore gemstones inside their breast-plates to safeguard them during battle.

The different healing properties of each type of crystal are believed to be based on the energy 'vibrations' they emit. The theory

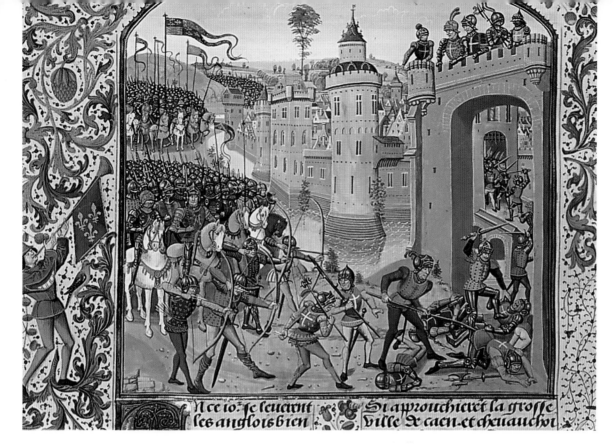

Edward III of England and his troops taking the French town of Caen in 1346. Medieval knights wore gemstones to protect them during battle.

Ice io: fe feuant Si approuchieret la groffe
fes anglois bien villé De caen et desuauchot

is that when you hold or wear a crystal, its natural energy field influences the energies of your body. Crystals can be easily obtained from speciality shops or from reputable gem dealers. For a listing of natural crystals and their various properties, turn to page 106.

Crystal Elixirs

The crystal's energies can also be captured in a water elixir made by placing a natural crystal in pure spring water and leaving it in bright sunlight for a given length of time until the liquid becomes imbued with the crystal's properties (see page 106). The elixirs can be added to the bath or made into spritzes to spray the skin. Their properties depend on the crystal chosen. Several of the crystal elixirs are said to have healing or restorative properties on the mind and body, such as those made with aquamarine, jasper and fluorite, while others, such as those made with clear quartz, rose quartz and sapphire, are thought to promote internal balance and feelings of harmony with nature.

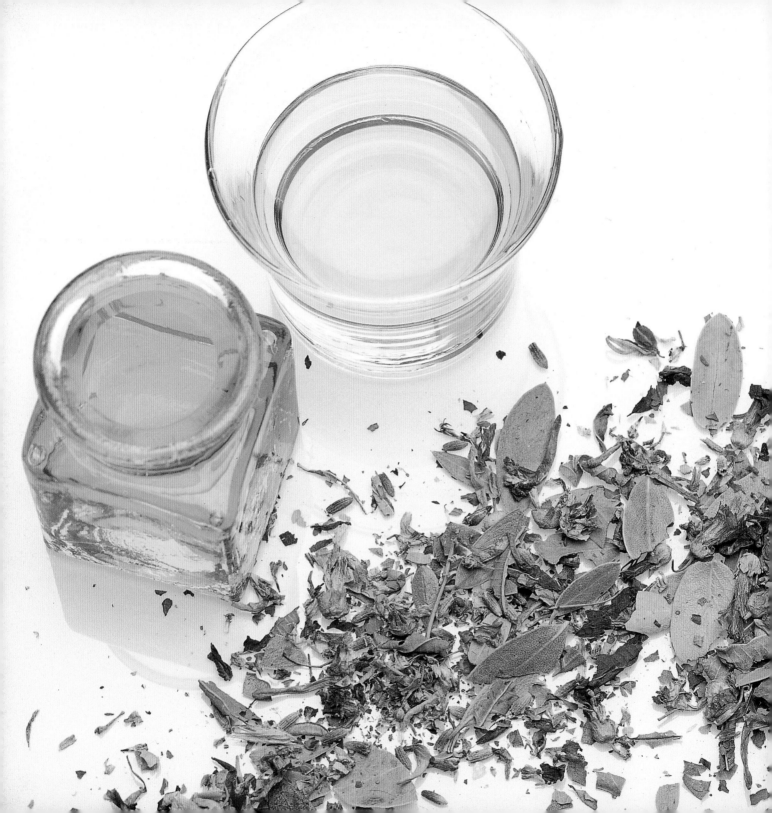

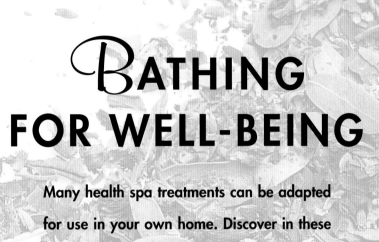

BATHING FOR WELL-BEING

Many health spa treatments can be adapted for use in your own home. Discover in these pages how water — used alone or in combination with therapeutic oils, herbs and minerals — can help to combat even the severe pain of rheumatism and arthritis, and alleviate debilitating skin conditions, such as eczema and psoriasis, allergies, colds and aching muscles, as well as enhancing your general health and well-being.

Decongestant baths

Next time you get a cold, don't snuffle and mope. Transform your bathroom into a healing sanctuary, try some decongestant treatments and start feeling better.

Colds can last from four to ten days. Flu is much more debilitating and can knock you out for at least two weeks. The stronger your immune system, the quicker you will shake off any virus infection. While you are suffering, though, there are plenty of ways to soothe discomfort and speed recovery. Warm decongestant baths are one way to alleviate symptoms and help to combat the virus.

Healing Herbal Baths

The best herbs to use in the bath are those that promote perspiration and speed the metabolism (as long as you also drink plenty of water to keep up your fluid levels). This helps your body to repel the virus more quickly. Herbs to use include the following (see A handful of herbs, pages 54–5 for ways to use them in your bath):

- **Fresh lemon balm** Good if you are feverish.
- **Yarrow** Warming and also improves the body's circulation. The leaves and blossom promote sweating. If your flu is severe, combine yarrow with elderflowers and peppermint and add some ginger (powdered or fresh).

Care for your face

Protect your forehead, cheeks and eyes with a towel when inhaling hot steam, to prevent swelling of the tiny blood vessels beneath the skin. Reduce puffiness around the eyes with an infusion of camomile, and use marsh mallow, elderflower or crushed strawberries to combat redness.

- **Peppermint** Stimulating and decongestant. Helps to clear mucus from nose and sinuses.
- **Elderflower** Helps to ease congestion from head, ears and chest. Can be combined with yarrow blossom and peppermint.
- **Sage** Helps to relieve muscular aches and pains and also eases congestion. Sage has antiseptic properties. **Caution** Avoid if pregnant.
- **Pine** Stimulates the skin to induce perspiration, but has a calming effect on the mind. You can obtain ready-prepared pine extract from a health food shop. This herb can be combined with lemon balm, elderflowers and peppermint leaves for increased effect. Avoid any product that contains artificial colourants.

Ease Your Cold

Congested Nose and Sinuses

Prepare a bowl of steaming hot water and add a few drops of eucalyptus, peppermint and lavender essential oils. Hot steam can scald and may also damage the mucus membrane in the nose, so wait until the steam is pleasantly warm. Hold your face over the bowl — at least 25cm (10in) away — and cover your head with a towel. Inhale the warm vapour for about five minutes (coming up for air when you feel too hot).

Fever

If you have a mild fever (about 38.5°C/101°F), drink plenty of fluids. A decongestant bath (warm — not hot) or cool sponge bath, will help to refresh the skin. However, always seek me— dical advice.

Warming, soothing and stimulating plants and oils, such as lavender, ginger, eucalyptus and pine, can reduce fever and relieve congestion, especially when combined with steam. Drink lots of water or herbal tea to replace fluids.

Soothe your aches and pains

Water is one of the most effective therapies for the treatment of severe aches and pains in chronic conditions such as rheumatism and arthritis.

There are numerous theories why some people develop rheumatism and arthritis; living in a damp climate, poor lymphatic circulation, too much stress, an over-acidic constitution, years of eating an imbalanced diet, for example. The list of potential triggers seems endless — and meaningless when you're in the middle of a particularly excruciating attack. For the majority of sufferers the main anti-dote is a powerful painkiller, often in several doses a day, to the point of nausea. Painkillers certainly dull the pain — initially at least. But as many sufferers discover after years on the same medication, dosages eventually need to be increased, and the condition may never really seem to improve. Not all is doom and gloom, however. Some alternative therapies have yielded excellent results.

Naturopathy

Thousands of sufferers have found that their condition substantially improved when they followed a rigid naturopathic diet, including the elimination of all dairy products, red meat, alcohol, caffeine and any acid-producing food or drink. Arthritis is thought to be aggravated by an acidic condition, and denying the body the opportunity to produce acid can help to reduce arthritis symptoms. Arthritis and rheumatic problems are unknown in countries that eat a vegetarian diet, comprising mainly alkaline fruits and vegetables. Consult your doctor, however, if you are thinking of embarking on a naturopathic regime.

Hydrotherapy

Hydrotherapy is one of the most well-established treatments for the symptoms of arthritis and rheumatic conditions. Many European spas, such as Karlovy Vary in the Czech Republic and Baden-Baden in Germany, are renowned for their water therapies. Thousands of sufferers find that spending a few weeks each year at one of these spas can help to control their symptoms for several months.

Hydrotherapy works on a number of levels. Certain natural spring waters contain minerals that help to alleviate pain and other symptoms. But hydrotherapy is also based on applying water in a way that soothes aching joints and inflammation of

Jacuzzis, whirlpools and other hydro-therapy baths are a feature of most spas. Pain can float away as water jets massage sore joints and inflamed tissues exactly where they need it.

the surrounding tissues. A visit to a health spa specialising in arthritis cures is worth investigating, or ask your doctor to advise a course of hydrotherapy in your locality. Meanwhile, try some of the basic techniques at home in your own bathroom.

Caution For safety — especially if you have mobility problems — fit your bath with handrails and use a nonslip bathmat. Install a plastic bath cushion or mattress for extra comfort. A walk-in shower with a sitting facility could be the most convenient option when getting into the bath is difficult.

Hot Baths For Aching Joints
The warmth brought to aching joints by a daily hot bath can help to alleviate pain.

Hot baths also induce perspiration, which aids the elimination of toxins. For some additional benefits, you can mix in some herbs (see Herbal detoxification, pages 30–1). Portable whirlpools are also extremely useful because the massaging action of the water, in combination with its warmth, is very soothing to the joints.

Inflammation
Cold poultices and cold-water treatments can help reduce inflammation. Make a poultice, using cold water on a cloth, and apply to the inflamed area.

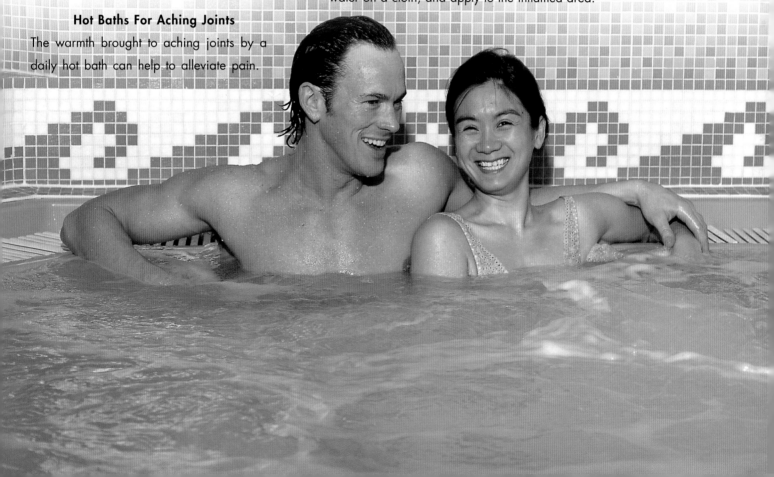

After-exercise restoratives

Gentle stretching before and after vigorous activity and completing your workout with a warm shower and massage, keeps your muscles supple and makes sure that exercise really does keep you fit.

Exercise induces the build-up of lactic acid in the muscles, which is why a cool-down stretch is important to help disperse it. Without this precaution, your muscles are likely to become stiff and uncomfortable. Usually some gentle stretching, followed by a relaxing hot shower or bath and massage, is all you need to ease slight discomfort away. When muscles are tired, and when they feel more strained than usual, there are a number of therapeutic baths that can help.

Are You Overdoing It?

Exercise can sometimes feel so invigorating that you get carried away and do too much. It promotes the production of 'feel good' chemicals (endorphins) in the brain. As you extend your activity, they can make you feel increasingly elated. They also act as natural painkillers, so that you may not realise you are pushing yourself too far.

Minimising the risks Never exercise without warming your muscles beforehand by gentle stretching or running on the spot. Do the kind of exercise that is right for you; for example, if you have weak knees, jogging is not a good idea. Most importantly, always stop exercising at the first sign of pain.

Over-exerting yourself puts too much stress on the muscles and can lead to injury. When muscle strain after exercise feels more severe than usual, you may have literally overstretched yourself.

Muscle Relief

Mineral salts, such as magnesium and potassium, have a relaxing effect and help to prevent cramp. Add 500g (1lb) of Epsom salts to the bathwater. Sprinkle in a couple of drops of rosemary essential oil (diluted in carrier oil). Soak for 20 minutes.

Cider vinegar restorer Add a cup of cider vinegar to the hot water. Massage weary muscles while you have a good soak in the bath.

Whirlpool baths are available in some health clubs, gyms and spas. The action of the water stimulates the flow of blood to overworked muscles and relaxes them, while its rotatory movement has an analgesic (painkilling) effect.

Water treatments and a soothing massage can help tired and strained muscles. Massage is most beneficial when the muscles are relaxed by a warm shower or a bath infused with restoring ingredients.

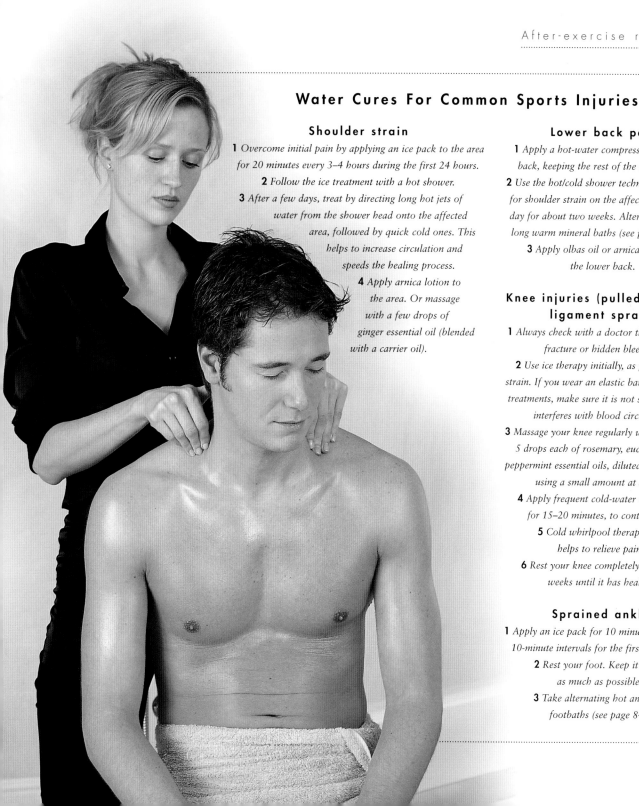

Water Cures For Common Sports Injuries

Shoulder strain

1 *Overcome initial pain by applying an ice pack to the area for 20 minutes every 3–4 hours during the first 24 hours.*
2 *Follow the ice treatment with a hot shower.*
3 *After a few days, treat by directing long hot jets of water from the shower head onto the affected area, followed by quick cold ones. This helps to increase circulation and speeds the healing process.*
4 *Apply arnica lotion to the area. Or massage with a few drops of ginger essential oil (blended with a carrier oil).*

Lower back pain

1 *Apply a hot-water compress to the lower back, keeping the rest of the body warm.*
2 *Use the hot/cold shower technique described for shoulder strain on the affected area every day for about two weeks. Alternate this with long warm mineral baths (see pages 40–41).*
3 *Apply olbas oil or arnica cream to the lower back.*

Knee injuries (pulled muscles, ligament sprain)

1 *Always check with a doctor that there is no fracture or hidden bleeding.*
2 *Use ice therapy initially, as for shoulder strain. If you wear an elastic bandage between treatments, make sure it is not so tight that it interferes with blood circulation.*
3 *Massage your knee regularly with a blend of 5 drops each of rosemary, eucalyptus and peppermint essential oils, diluted in carrier oil, using a small amount at a time.*
4 *Apply frequent cold-water compresses for 15–20 minutes, to control pain.*
5 *Cold whirlpool therapy also helps to relieve pain.*
6 *Rest your knee completely for a few weeks until it has healed.*

Sprained ankle

1 *Apply an ice pack for 10 minutes. Repeat at 10-minute intervals for the first few hours.*
2 *Rest your foot. Keep it raised as much as possible.*
3 *Take alternating hot and cold footbaths (see page 84).*

Improve your circulation

Simple hydrotherapy techniques for use at home can give your circulation a boost, improve your overall health and light your skin with the glow of well-being.

A healthy lifestyle is the best way to maintain good circulation. But there are additional ways to boost a sluggish system. Hydrotherapy provides some of the most effective techniques and there are a variety of baths you can take to relieve circulatory problems.

Rosemary bath For a general improvement in circulation take regular baths infused with rosemary solution (see pages 30–31). You can complement the herbs with 3–4 drops of rosemary essential oil (blended in a carrier oil) in the bathwater. Before

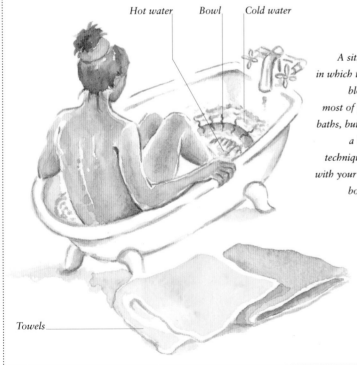

Hot water   Bowl   Cold water

Towels

Sitz bath

A sitz bath (from the German word for sitting) is a water therapy technique in which the thighs and pelvic area only are submerged in a shallow bath. It improves blood circulation in those areas, which is especially useful if you spend most of your days seated (at a desk, for example). Spas have specially designed sitz baths, but any basin, bath or bidet, of suitable size, can be used. Immerse your feet in a bowl of hot water at the same time for additional benefit. Adapt the technique to your regular bath by sitting in shallow water (about 15cm/6in deep), with your knees bent, or your legs propped over the side of the bath. Keep your upper body and legs warm with towels. Vary the temperature of the sitz bath according to the required effect.

• Cold water helps congestion in the intestinal region. Spend about 10 seconds to 2 minutes in the bath.
• A warm sitz bath can relieve cramps and spasms and is useful for alleviating period pain. Stay in the bath for 5–15 minutes.
• A contrasting sitz bath — switching from warm to cold two or three times — is beneficial for bladder and kidney conditions and in treating pelvic congestion generally.

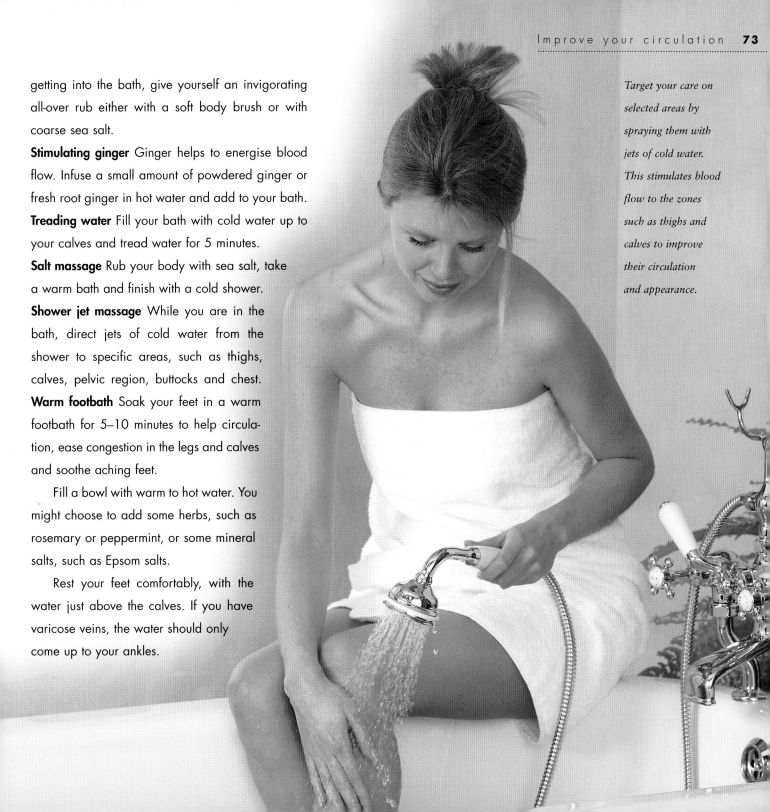

getting into the bath, give yourself an invigorating all-over rub either with a soft body brush or with coarse sea salt.

Stimulating ginger Ginger helps to energise blood flow. Infuse a small amount of powdered ginger or fresh root ginger in hot water and add to your bath.

Treading water Fill your bath with cold water up to your calves and tread water for 5 minutes.

Salt massage Rub your body with sea salt, take a warm bath and finish with a cold shower.

Shower jet massage While you are in the bath, direct jets of cold water from the shower to specific areas, such as thighs, calves, pelvic region, buttocks and chest.

Warm footbath Soak your feet in a warm footbath for 5–10 minutes to help circulation, ease congestion in the legs and calves and soothe aching feet.

Fill a bowl with warm to hot water. You might choose to add some herbs, such as rosemary or peppermint, or some mineral salts, such as Epsom salts.

Rest your feet comfortably, with the water just above the calves. If you have varicose veins, the water should only come up to your ankles.

Target your care on selected areas by spraying them with jets of cold water. This stimulates blood flow to the zones such as thighs and calves to improve their circulation and appearance.

Treatments for skin problems

Skin conditions, such as eczema, psoriasis and acne, can flare up for a variety of complex reasons. But there are natural remedies that can help to alleviate them.

There are many theories why some people are more prone to skin problems than others. Eczema, psoriasis and acne may be triggered by allergies, emotional stress, hormonal imbalance, toxic overload or hereditary predisposition.

The conventional Western approach is to deal with the symptoms through the application of creams or by internal medication. The Chinese way, which is noted for some striking results in treating skin disorders, views symptoms as the sign of an imbalance that needs to be adjusted. A Chinese doctor would first seek to find out where the imbalance in the body lies, and then prescribe herbs to remedy it.

Whichever route you take towards a cure, however, symptoms such as itchy, weeping, scaly skin or painful spots and boils can be extremely distressing. There are a number of self-help tactics which can help to alleviate — and sometimes even eliminate — the worst of these symptoms. A therapeutic bath with skin-soothing and calming ingredients is often an immediately helpful treatment.

Soothing Facial Skin

Soothe irritated facial skin by applying organic seaweed directly, or make a face pack with seaweed powder and warm water. The leaves or extract of aloe vera can help heal broken skin. A face pack mixed from bran and warm water or yoghurt can calm inflammation.

◀ *Oak bark, bran and natural oils, such as evening primrose and borage, are among the substances that have proved beneficial in easing itching and reducing the severity of skin problems.*

Skin-soothing Baths

Eczema

A warm bath, with added camomile (see pages 54–5) will help to calm itchy or weeping skin. An alternative is a solution containing calendula flowers, chickweed, oak bark, bran or walnut leaves.

Hives

Hives are characterised by raised, itchy, weal-like patches that come up suddenly — possibly in response to anxiety or food sensitivity. A bath containing bran may help to reduce the inflammation. Bring 110g (4oz) of bran in water to the boil. Cool slightly, and add to the bath. Oats are also soothing. Place them in a cheesecloth or muslin bag and attach to the tap, so that the hot water runs through them. You can also use a mixture of oats and bran (2:1 ratio) in both cases.

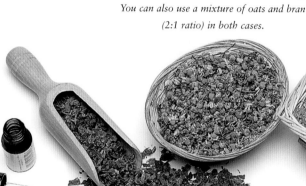

Psoriasis

Typical symptoms include dry, scaly skin that flakes off and causes intense irritation. Hot water can aggravate the condition, so stick to brief warm baths. Avoid soap, which can also irritate. Dead Sea salt (see pages 40–41) can reduce the itching greatly. Add 1.8kg (4lb) to your bath. Finish with a cool shower. Use water saturated with sea salt to make a soothing compress. Sea water and a reasonable amount of sunshine are extremely beneficial.

- *Avoid acid-forming foods such as dairy products, meat, wheat and citrus fruits (except for lemons).*
- *Practise stress-reduction techniques, for example, meditation, visualisation or yoga. Psoriasis tends to worsen with stress.*

Acne

Acne is not just the badly timed arrival of a pimple or two, but a full-blown eruption of pimples, resulting from inflammation of the sebaceous glands.

- *Add camomile or calendula to your bath to improve the general condition of your skin and prevent the formation of acne scars.*
- *Use rosemary and lavender essential oils, which are beneficial for all problem skin. Dilute 5–6 drops of either (or a mixture of the two) in a carrier oil and add to your bath (see Essential oils, pages 38–9).*
- *A course of Chinese herbs, prescribed to individual needs by a qualified practitioner, can help.*

A bath infused with the right natural ingredients for your condition, such as calendula and camomile (above), may be the best way to relieve immediate discomfort and begin the healing process.

THE HEALING POWERS OF SACRED WATERS

Water is revered in every culture and region of the world. It is an innate part of our being, fundamental to our survival, and frequently invested with supernatural powers of purification, healing and regeneration.

By cleansing their sins in the sacred Ganges, Hindus prepare for their return to joy in heaven.

TO THE EARLY CHRISTIANS, immersion in water during baptism was a symbol of spiritual purification; a cleansing ritual that marked initiation into a new life as a member of the Church. However, the concept of consecrated water predates Christianity, and plays a role in most other major religions. The thousands of Hindus who flock to bathe in the sacred River Ganges in India believe that a single day's bathing washes away the sins of many lifetimes and frees them from the eternal treadmill of reincarnation. Part of the reason why water is so central to religious devotion may be that water is integral to our very essence. The human body is 70 per cent water, and without it we die. In every creation story — from

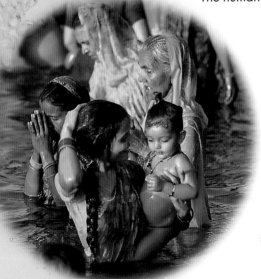

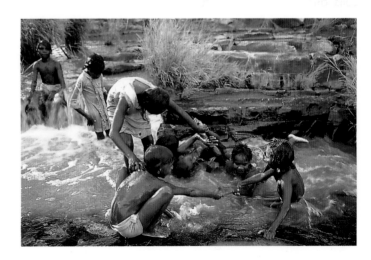

Many native Australian Aboriginal people regard water as the source of life.

the Christian *Genesis* to the sacred texts of the Hindus, from native Australian Aboriginal to native North American beliefs — water is the source of life. Water, as the element from which all living creatures emerged, was seen by these peoples as synonymous with life itself. It is not surprising, therefore, that water came also to symbolise spiritual rebirth in many cultures.

Source of Miracles

Water is also regarded as the great purifier; the cleanser of souls and bodies. In certain sacred places it is revered for its healing qualities. Natural springs have become the centre of local cults and the destination for religious pilgrimage. Perhaps the most famous in Europe is the spring water that emerges

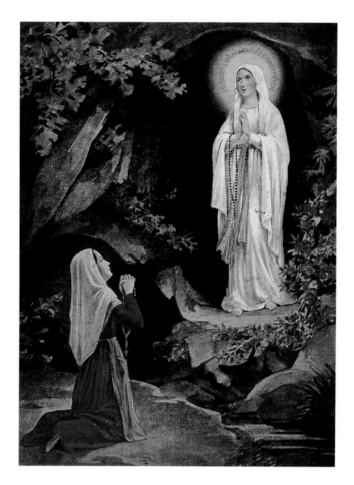

A traditional portrayal of the apparition of the Virgin Mary to Saint Bernadette at Lourdes in 1858. The healing spring that emerged at the time was found to be rich in a therapeutic mineral.

just outside the small town of Lourdes in southwest France, known for its miraculous healing powers. For more than a century pilgrims have made their way to the holy spring in their thousands, in search of cures for ailments of the mind, spirit and body, and even today people claim to have recovered from serious illnesses as a result of a visit to the mystical place. Although the many miraculous cures reported from Lourdes are generally seen as the manifestation of the power of faith and the direct intervention of Our Lady, scientists have discovered that the water contains an abundance of the mineral germanium, which is known to have a strong therapeutic effect on a number of degenerative diseases. Some natural springs in Japan are also rich in germanium and they too are considered sacred for their healing powers.

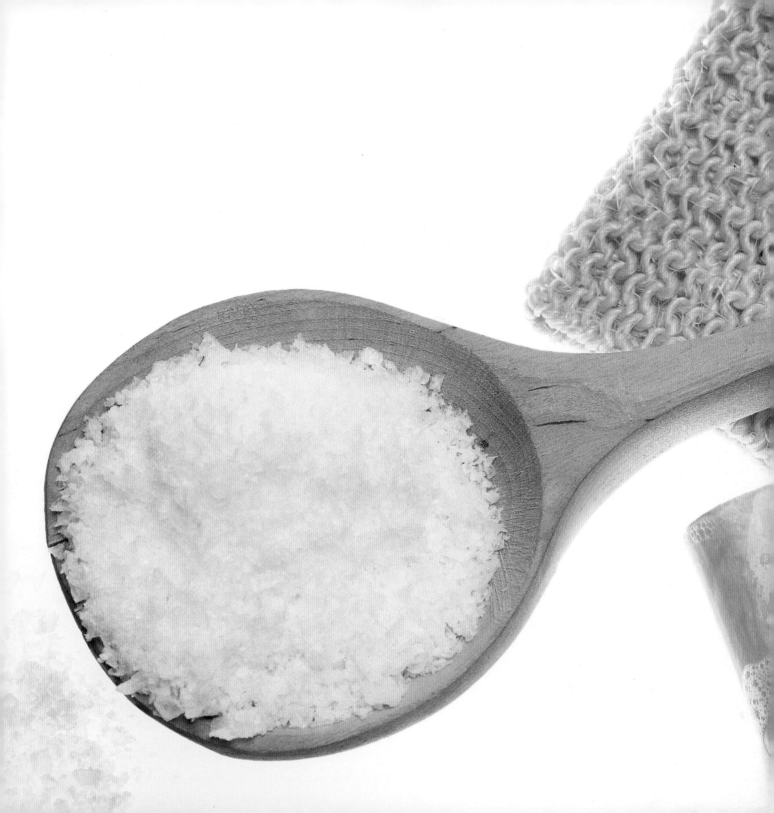

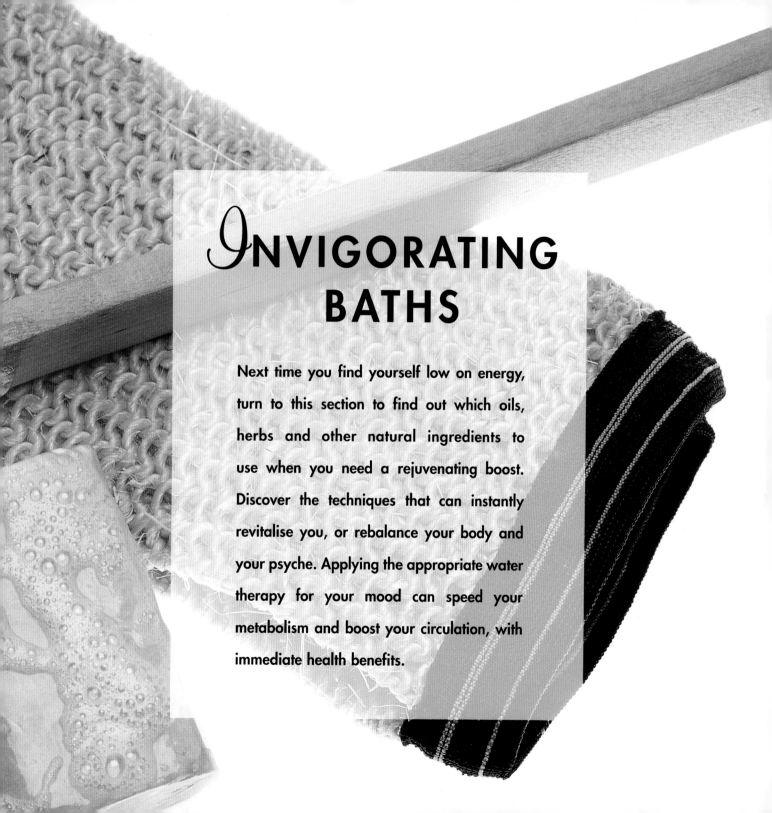

𝒥NVIGORATING BATHS

Next time you find yourself low on energy, turn to this section to find out which oils, herbs and other natural ingredients to use when you need a rejuvenating boost. Discover the techniques that can instantly revitalise you, or rebalance your body and your psyche. Applying the appropriate water therapy for your mood can speed your metabolism and boost your circulation, with immediate health benefits.

Revitalise!

It's normal at times for energy to hit a low ebb. But next time you feel tired, try a water treatment that will make you eager to get up and go.

Do you ever feel so drained that you can barely move? Does getting up in the morning sometimes feel like a major effort? When some work or event is coming up which is really important to you, but you can't get motivated — that's when you need an invigorating bath. Forget the idea of a hot steaming soak, which will make you want to go back to sleep again. Opt for one of these energy-boosting treatments.

The Classic Cold Shower

A cold shower is a foolproof way to galvanise your system. And it need not be torture. Rub yourself briskly with a soft body brush or hemp glove first, and begin with a warm shower. Then just as you are beginning to warm up, switch the temperature to cold gradually. Spray your entire body for 30–60 seconds. Then dry yourself vigorously with a towel.

▶ *Enhance the effect of the bracing herbs in your bath by an all-over rub with a sisal friction mitt.*

Salt Rub

Enhance the effect of a herbal bath by giving yourself a salt massage beforehand. Make a paste of coarse salt granules or sea salt, mixed with warm water, and massage it in a circular motion all over your body, using your hands or a sisal friction mitt. The salt helps to boost circulation and tone the skin. Do this for a few minutes and then slip into your herbal bath. Round off your bath by splashing yourself with cold water and rubbing yourself dry with a coarse towel.
***Caution** Do not apply salt if you have any broken skin.*

A salt treatment can make your bath as invigorating as a dip in the ocean.

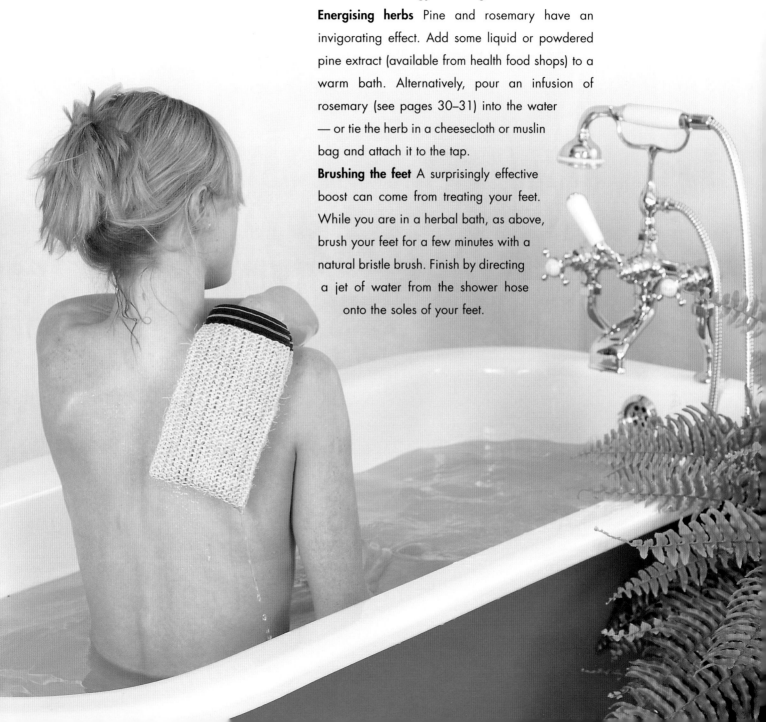

Energy-boosting Baths

Energising herbs Pine and rosemary have an invigorating effect. Add some liquid or powdered pine extract (available from health food shops) to a warm bath. Alternatively, pour an infusion of rosemary (see pages 30–31) into the water — or tie the herb in a cheesecloth or muslin bag and attach it to the tap.

Brushing the feet A surprisingly effective boost can come from treating your feet. While you are in a herbal bath, as above, brush your feet for a few minutes with a natural bristle brush. Finish by directing a jet of water from the shower hose onto the soles of your feet.

Enlivening oils

A few drops of stimulating essential oil added to your bath or shower can make all the difference to your energy levels.

Energising Oils to Use in the Bath

Essential oil	Characteristics	Effects
Cardamom	*Warming, spicy, oriental*	*Helps dispel mental fatigue. Calms indigestion and stomach cramps.*
Cinnamon	*Spicy, woody*	*Restorative. Combats fatigue. Good for poor circulation, spasms, cramps and sluggish digestion.*
Clove[1]	*Spicy, oriental*	*Reinvigorating and cleansing. Helpful for rheumatic pains, asthma and bronchitis.*
Lemon	*Light, fruity*	*Revives mental clarity. Good for sore throats, poor circulation and cellulite.*
Grapefruit	*Fruity, citrus*	*Invigorating, refreshing, cleansing. Helpful for water retention, acne, muscle fatigue and general stiffness.*
Sweet orange	*Citrus, sweet*	*Uplifting and reviving, a tonic to the nervous system. Good for stress.*
Mandarin	*Sweet, warm, fruity*	*Soothing and uplifting. Helps skin problems, stretch marks and fluid retention.*
Bergamot	*Sweet, light, citrus*	*Refreshing, reviving, antidepressant. Calms the nervous system and re-energises. Good for flu, colds and skin problems.*
Rosemary[2]	*Fresh and woody*	*Purifying and restorative. Very stimulating. Aids the metabolism and circulation. Helps reduce fluid retention and muscular pain.*
Sandalwood	*Woody, balsamic*	*Balances the nervous system and is physically uplifting. Useful in depression, nervous disorders, acne, catarrh and problem skin.*
Peppermint[3]	*Fresh, minty*	*Energising. Clears the mind. Good for muscular aches and stomach cramps.*

Caution: 1 *Can irritate sensitive skins.* **2** *Do not use if pregnant.* **3** *Do not use if taking homeopathic remedies. Mint has an antidote effect.*

Essential oils can induce a variety of moods and responses, depending upon their key chemical constituents. These chemicals act on the brain and the nervous system to promote specific effects. The proportions of its components are what gives an oil its essential 'character'. Oils from the chemical group known as esters, for example, induce a soothing, sedative reaction. They are useful if you are feeling over-stressed and want to be gently refreshed.

Stimulating Oils

Oils that are high in phenols on the other hand, for example peppermint, are much more stimulating. So it's worth keeping a few of these handy for occasions when you feel yourself flagging. Add them to your bath, or use an essential oil cleansing gel in the shower. **Caution** Do not use citrus oils on the skin before going out in bright sunlight, because they could trigger a phototoxic reaction. Never apply essential oils directly to your skin. Always dilute in bathwater or in a carrier oil: about 5ml (1 tsp) carrier oil per 1 drop essential oil. Use 3–6 drops of oil per bath. (See Essential oils, pages 38–9.) Once mixed, keep refrigerated and use within three months.

Combine a refreshing shower with the restorative effect of a cleansing gel that contains one of the recommended stimulating oils.

Hot or cold — or both?

Varying the temperature of your bath or shower can bring important benefits.

Whether you bath in hot, cold or warm water does make a difference.

When you want to relax, a long hot bath is the answer. Warm water increases the flow of blood to the skin. Cold water, on the other hand, constricts the blood vessels and firms your skin. As soon as you leave the cold water, blood flows back to make you feel uniquely revitalised. Switching from hot water to cold feels invigorating, boosts your energy and can fortify the system generally.

Shallow Hot Bath

Taking a quick, shallow, hot bath can ease problems centred around the pelvic area by bringing blood selectively to that part of the body. It helps to get the colon moving, decrease menstrual cramps, reduce discomfort in the lower back and can alleviate the painful symptoms of cystitis.

Bathing in Cold Water

Cold baths and showers are a feature of many spas. They are thought to improve circulation and even increase resistance to disease. However, there are a few cautions to bear in mind before taking the plunge, for health and comfort reasons.

Cold-water safety Do not bath in cold water if you suffer from high blood pressure, heart disease or any major health problem.

From hot to cold Always warm your body before taking the plunge. Take a sauna or a warm bath first, or at least heat yourself from the inside by drinking a warming herbal tea. Then, while you still feel warm all over, step into the cold bath or shower. After the initial shock, the water will begin to feel almost warm. Do not stay longer than a minute or two and dry yourself energetically.

A Hot and Cold Footbath

A footbath is wonderfully refreshing, and is useful for treating sprains. Place your feet in a bowl of hot

> ### Clear Your Head —
> ### By Treating Your Feet
>
> *If your head feels congested, apply a jet of cold water from the shower directly onto the soles of your feet. This is thought to work because reflex points on the feet are linked to major organs and body parts.*

Hands are exposed continually to the rigours of work and the environment — and are always on display. Improve blood flow and counter cold-weather damage by giving them an alternate hot and cold water treatment.

water for 3 minutes. Then plunge them into cold water for 30 seconds. Repeat three times. Usually a footbath ends with cold water, but if you are treating a sprained ankle, finish with the hot footbath. Add a few drops of lavender essential oil to the water to enhance the therapeutic effect.

Alternate Hot and Cold Showers

Switching from hot to cold water is very easy in the shower. Turn on the spray for 15 seconds hot, followed by 15 seconds cold water.

Hot and Cold Hand Baths

This is a useful self-treatment to improve the circulation to your hands. It is a good remedy for chilblains and wrist strain. Prepare a bowl each of hot and cold water. Submerge your hands in the hot water for 3 minutes, and in the cold water for half a minute. Repeat three times.

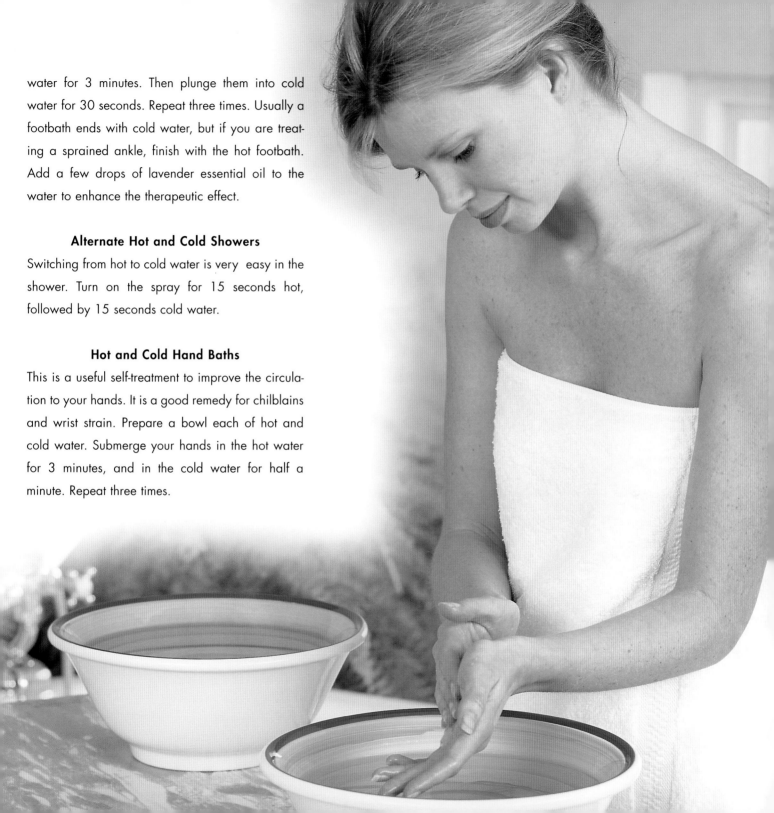

JAPANESE BATHS

The Japanese have made bathing almost an art form — whether at home, in the bathhouse or in the wealth of hot springs with which their country abounds.

BATHING HAS ALWAYS FIGURED PROMINENTLY in Japanese culture. According to the Shinto religion, physical cleanliness is of utmost importance, because it symbolises purity and virtue. It may seem surprising, therefore, that most Japanese homes acquired a bathroom only in the last 20 or 30 years. Until then, the popular practice was to visit hot springs or the public bathhouse — usually as a family.

Bathing in the hot spring at Nagano — one of the many in Japan — provides the twin pleasures of natural water and fresh air.

Public bathhouses, or *sento*, began to make an appearance in the 16th and 17th centuries. They were immediately popular, since, in addition to providing washing facilities, they also became a focal point of

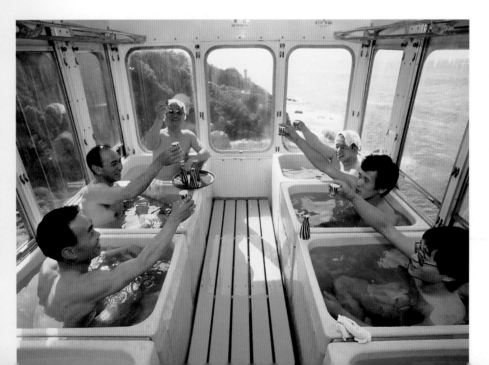

The perfect way to socialise: in the hot bath of a cable car high above Wakayama, drinking sake with friends.

Japanese social life. For a long time mixed bathing was the norm, but the influx of visitors from Europe and America in the 19th century prompted legislation to ban this practice. Modern bathhouses retain many of the old-style features; an anteroom for removing shoes, a dressing room, a relaxation area for reading and taking refreshments, a vast tiled bathing area lined with showers, taps, and several hot and cold water baths to soak in.

Japan's *Onsen*

The Japanese value their natural hot mineral springs, known as *onsen*, for their therapeutic properties, and thousands visit them throughout the year. The acid *onsen* at Kusatsu, Nasu and Yumoto, are said to relieve skin conditions, venereal diseases and rheumatism. The carbon-dioxydated *onsen* at Arima, north of Kobe, are renowned for their therapeutic effects on conditions such as heart disease, neuralgia and high blood pressure. The Beppu *onsen*, on Japan's southern island of Kyushu, are popular because the waters contain almost every kind of mineral. Bathing in these hot springs, surrounded by nature in the open air, is truly an experience to remember.

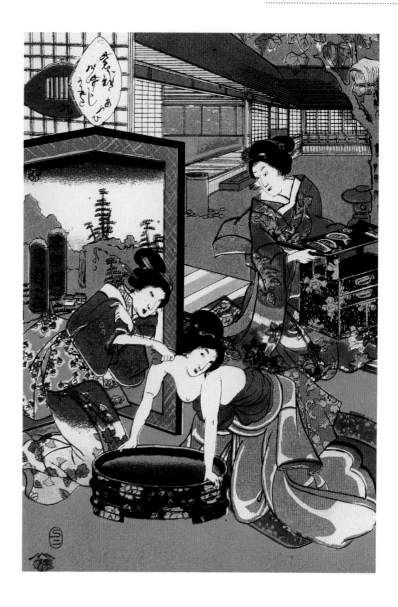

A 19th-century woodblock print of a Japanese lady at her toilet.

Whether bathing at home, in a public bathhouse or hot spring, the Japanese always wash carefully with soap and an exfoliating cloth and rinse before entering the water. To use soap in the water is unthinkable as it is only for soaking in and is shared with other bathers. At home, the Japanese often add therapeutic bath products, such as mineral salts and herbs, to leave the skin silky and soft.

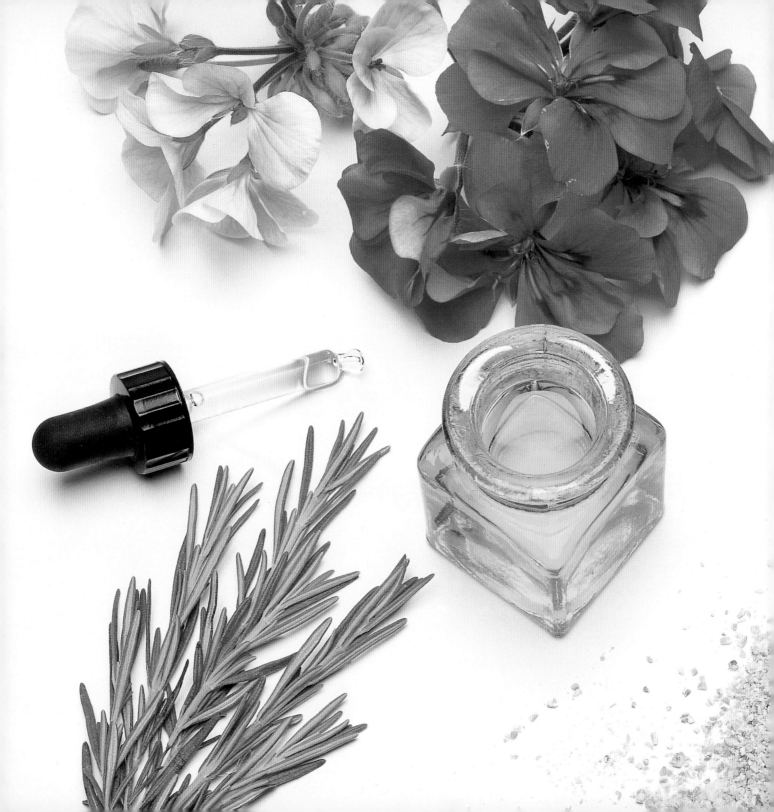

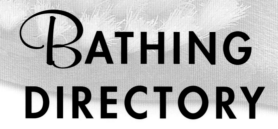

BATHING DIRECTORY

This section gives you recipes and tips for baths and treatments to soothe, vitalise and beautify. Helpful information about plants, oils, minerals, cosmetic ingredients, spa therapies and where to enjoy them will help you get the most from your bathing.

Body care

All of us tend to ignore our skin and bodies — especially during the winter months when we wear winter clothes. We pay the price for this neglect when warmer weather or a looming holiday inspires us to don shorts and swimsuits.

You can feel confident about your body's appearance all year-round if you use your bathtime as an opportunity to deal with 'problem areas' before they are a problem! Practising some of the body-care treatments that follow can help to revitalise the look of your skin and hair.

Drink 1.2 litres (2 pints) of water each day.

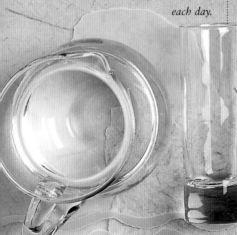

Drink Regularly

When you exercise — especially in hot weather — check that you are drinking enough water and other fluids.

- *Heat makes you sweat more (a function of the body's cooling system), and you need to replace fluid more frequently. When you lose more than 3 per cent of your body weight in fluid, you begin to tire more easily. And over 5 per cent puts you at serious risk of heatstroke.*
- *Thirst is the best indicator that you are losing fluids. But keep in mind that by the time you begin to feel thirsty, you are already getting dehydrated. So drink water at regular intervals while you exercise; every 20–30 minutes when doing moderate exercise, and every 15 minutes when exercise is more intense, or when considerable endurance is called for.*

Cellulite

Lumpy orange-peel skin tends to affect women more than men. It appears mostly on hips and thighs, although its distinctive puckered and dimpled appearance is not unknown on the stomach, knees and upper arms. These nodular pockets of fat are caused primarily by poor circulation, which inhibits the elimination of fluid and toxins.

It is notoriously difficult to shift — but not impossible. Try the following treatments for a marked improvement:

- A weekly sauna eliminates about 30 per cent of toxins through the pores (see pages 26–7).

Exfoliate by skin brushing with sea salt.

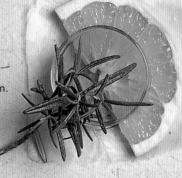

Boost your circulation with grapefruit and rosemary oil.

- Grapefruit and rosemary essential oils have properties that stimulate circulation. Add a few drops, diluted in a carrier oil, to your bath (see Essential oils, pages 38–9).
- Improve the texture of your skin by rubbing in sea salt lightly with a coarse body mitt (see Skin brushing, pages 14–15).
- Apply some hydrotherapy. Use the shower spray to direct a jet of warm water over the affected areas to stimulate the blood vessels.
- Massage the skin with either vitamin E oil, almond or apricot oil after bathing. This will help to boost circulation and improve skin texture.

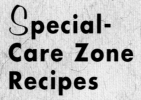

Hands are a special-care zone.

- Exercise also diminishes stress, which promotes the formation of cellulite by disrupting hormone levels. Enhance the effect with regular de-stressing baths — see the Relaxing Baths section, pages 48–63 for some suitable, soothing soaks.
- Also recommended is using the recipe for 'Strawberry and Ginger Reviver', see right, once or twice a week.

Strawberries, ginger and kaolin clay powder blended together will work wonders for circulation.

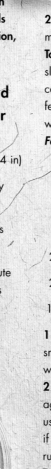

Special-Care Zone Recipes

The following recipes are for treatments that will help with cellulite, as well as the hands and feet. For more information, see left and pages 22–3.

Strawberry and Ginger Reviver

YOU WILL NEED

1 ginger root, about 10cm (4 in)

2 tbsp (30ml) kaolin clay powder

7 or 8 large strawberries

1 Put all ingredients into a blender and whiz for a minute or so, until the ginger is puréed with the other ingredients.

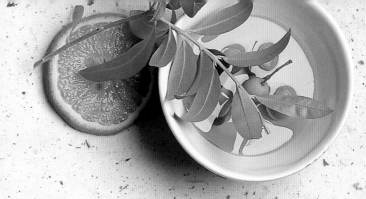

2 If the mix is too runny, add more kaolin clay powder.

To use Apply onto areas with sluggish circulation and/or cellulite and leave to dry for a few minutes. Rinse with cool water and pat the skin dry.

For external use only

Foot Rub Lotion

YOU WILL NEED

2 tbsp (30ml) of cocoa butter

2 tsp (10ml) calendula tincture

2 tbsp (30ml) calendula petals

1 tbsp (15ml) camomile flowers

1 Heat the cocoa butter in a small bowl over simmering water, then mix in the tincture.
2 Add the flowers and mix again vigorously. You can use a blender but it may clog if the cocoa butter is not runny enough.

To use Rub the fresh mixture into the feet, especially the soles of the feet, concentrating on the reflexology points.

Orange essential oil and olive oil are excellent skin conditioners.

Olive Oil Hand Conditioner

YOU WILL NEED

2 tbsp (30ml) olive oil

2 drops orange essential oil

1 drop frankincense essential oil

1 Mix the oils together in a small bowl.
2 Decant into a bottle that has a secure lid and store in the refrigerator.

To use This is especially good as an overnight treatment to give very dry hands, or eczema patches, a chance to heal. Firstly, immerse your hands in the oil and get someone to help you put on thin plastic gloves. Sleep with the treatment and the gloves on. In the morning, rinse thoroughly and massage excess oil into hands.

For external use only

Bath Recipes

The following recipes can all be used to make natural therapeutic remedies. Some can be incorporated into your bathing routine, others are for specific conditions or skin types. When your body needs revitalising and reconditioning, treat yourself to one of these special bath recipes.

Therapeutic Seaweed Bath
YOU WILL NEED

1 sachet OR ½ cup (60g/2oz) seaweed powder (from a health shop)

1 drop rosemary and/or 1 drop lavender essential oil

1 tsp (5ml) almond oil

1 Run a warm bath and add the seaweed sachet or powder.
2 Blend and add the almond and essential oil(s).
3 Sit in the bath for 20 minutes.
4 Rinse off the residue with clean, warm water.

A cheesecloth or muslin sachet full of herbs, such as calendula and lavender leaves.

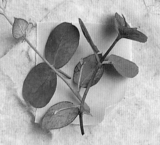

A Moisturising Herbal Bath
YOU WILL NEED

100g (3oz) of herbs

1.8 litres (3pts) of water

1 Put the herbs in a non-metallic pan, add the water and simmer for 15–20 minutes.
2 Strain, and add the liquid to the bath. For maximum effect, soak in the bath for about 20 minutes.
3 Use any discarded herbs as a scrub; tie them in a piece of cheesecloth or muslin, and rub them all over your skin. Choose a single herb or blend a combination.
4 Complement your herbal bath with a few drops of rose, lavender, neroli or jasmine essential oils (see Essential oils, pages 38–9) in the water.

Decongestant Bath
YOU WILL NEED

3 drops of eucalyptus oil

3 drops peppermint oil

3 drops lavender oil

A handful of steeped thyme or elderflowers (optional).

1 tbsp (15ml) carrier oil such as apricot kernel or almond

1 Mix ingredients and add to a hot bath.

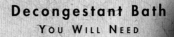

Eucalyptus and peppermint.

Cleopatra's Milk Bath
YOU WILL NEED

500g (1lb) dried non-fat milk powder

3–6 drops essential oil (diluted in a carrier oil).

1 Blend the milk powder with water until smooth, and add to your bath. Mix in the oil.

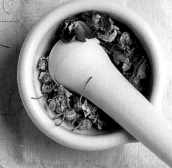

Flower petals and herbs can be ground with a pestle and mortar.

Herbal Bath Oil
YOU WILL NEED

8 tbsp (120ml) dried herbs ground to powder

2 tbsp (30ml) vodka or wine vinegar

Corn, safflower or olive oil

Medium-sized screwtop jar

Sieve

1 Pound 4 tbsp (60ml) herbs to a powder with a pestle and mortar.
2 Tip them into the jar, mix in the vodka or vinegar, and add the oil. Don't fill to the top.
3 Screw on the lid and place on a shelf that is exposed to sunlight. Leave for three weeks.
4 Strain the oil to remove the herb residue and add 4 tbsp (60ml) of powdered herbs. Leave for another three weeks.
5 Sieve the oil into a dark glass container. Store in a dark place.
6 Use as a therapeutic bath oil.
For external use only

Body Recipes

Body wraps and packs using natural ingredients such as mud and mustard are good for relaxing the body and relieving aching joints. (See Glorious mud, pages 42–3.)

Rose and Geranium Liquid Soap

YOU WILL NEED

1 tbsp (15ml) rose water

2 tbsp (30 ml) baking soda

2 drops rose oil

2 drops geranium oil

2 tbsp (30ml) aloe vera gel

1 Warm the rose water and dissolve the baking soda in it.
2 Cool until lukewarm, then add the essential oils. (Ensure that you don't add the essential oils before as they will evaporate.)
3 Fold in the aloe vera gel and refrigerate overnight to chill the mix completely.
4 Decant into a pump-top dispenser bottle for easy access. This soap is ideal for dry skin.
For external use only

Apricot Kernel Rough Skin Remover

YOU WILL NEED

2 tbsp (30ml) apricot kernels

2 tbsp (30 ml) rice bran

1 tsp (5ml) apricot kernel oil

1 Whiz the apricot kernels in a blender until ground finely.
2 Mix the ground kernels with the rice bran.
3 Mix in enough oil to just form a paste. It should be a thick, non-runny consistency.
4 Take a small amount in the palm of damp, clean hands. Rub into the rough skin areas, such as callouses on hands or rough patches on the feet, and rinse. Remember to use a gentle circular motion when using exfoliators.

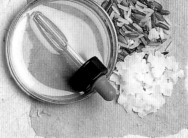
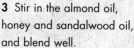

Apricot oil, kernels and rice.

Mud Body Pack

YOU WILL NEED

180g (6oz) Fuller's earth powder

1 cup (250ml/8fl oz) lemon or lime juice

2 tsp (10ml) almond oil

1 tsp (5ml) clear honey

1 drop sandalwood essential oil

1 For maximum benefit, 'prime' your body by exfoliating the skin.
2 Mix the mud or Fuller's earth into a thick paste with the lemon or lime juice. Add enough warm water to warm and liquefy the mixture.

Baking soda, aloe vera gel and rose oil and water.

3 Stir in the almond oil, honey and sandalwood oil, and blend well.
4 Spread the mixture over your entire body, starting with your feet. Ask a partner to do the parts of your back and middle shoulders that you cannot reach. If this is not possible, just focus on specific areas; thighs, to boost circulation and treat cellulite; and arms, legs or back for problem skin.
5 Cover the coated areas in plastic wrap or foil to retain the heat generated by the mud or clay.
6 Leave on for 15–20 minutes, then shower off under tepid water. Follow with a warm bath infused with a few drops of almond oil.
7 Drink plenty of water afterwards to rehydrate.

Lemon, lime and Fuller's earth powder.

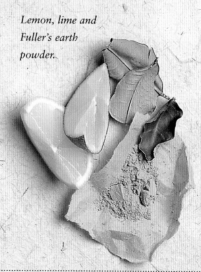

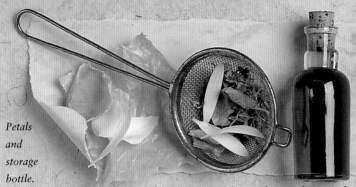

Petals and storage bottle.

Mustard Pack

YOU WILL NEED

1–2 tbsp (15–30ml) powdered mustard

6–8 tbsp (90–120ml) flour

Tepid water

Thick cloth or towel

1 Mix mustard and flour into a paste with tepid water.
2 Place in a folded cloth and heat by placing on a hot radiator or hot-water bottle.
3 Apply the pack to the painful joint. This helps bring blood to the surface of the skin, increasing circulation.
For external use only

Mustard powder, flour and natural cloth.

Floral Body Oil

YOU WILL NEED

Petals

Oil

Sieve

Storage bottle

1 Add as many petals as you can to a small pan of warmed oil (enough to fill your bottle).
2 Warm the oil by placing the pan in a larger pan of hot water. Leave on a very low heat for about two hours.
3 Sieve the oil to remove the petals, add a fresh supply. Repeat the process.
4 Sieve the final batch and decant into a bottle when cooled.
5 Store in a dark place. Use the oil within a few months.
For external use only

Water Aerobics

Water aerobics sessions are a feature at many spas and leisure centres. The natural buoyancy of water makes it much easier to do exercises that can seem tough in a regular aerobics class. Suddenly you can kick your legs much higher, and get into positions that would be impossible on dry land. The water supports your body, so that the exercises feel almost effortless — yet they are still effective. They help to tone your muscles, improve your flexibility and provide a cardiovascular workout. Even if you are not at a spa, you can try the following simple exercises at your local swimming pool.

Preparation

Warm up first by swimming a few lengths of the pool. If you are using an outdoor pool, remember to wear waterproof sunscreen.

To tone waist and hips

Make sure that the water level is between your stomach and shoulders. Stand close to the poolside with your hands gripping the edge, elbows pointed downwards and feet together. Slowly, so that you cannot really feel the resistance of the water, swing your whole body outwards to the right, as far up as you can, keeping your legs as straight as possible — like a pendulum. Come slowly back to your starting position. Repeat 10 times. Do the exercise 10 times again, but this time swinging to the left.

To tone thighs

Tread water for 2–3 minutes. Finish off and cool down by swimming two lengths of the pool.

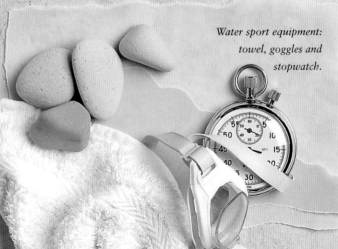

Water sport equipment: towel, goggles and stopwatch.

Hair Recipes

Washing and conditioning your hair with natural ingredients is preferable to bombarding it with chemicals. It would be difficult, however, to concoct an effective and practical shampoo without using a detergent.

All detergents are synthetically produced and therefore contain chemicals — even the supposedly more 'natural' ones, such as sodium lauryl sulphate (derived from coconut and palm oils).

A sensitive scalp is especially at risk, because detergents can aggravate skin conditions, including dermatitis and eczema. To safeguard your skin while

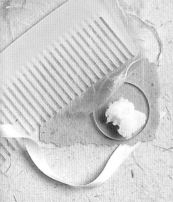

keeping your hair clean, choose shampoos that contain mild detergents — also called cleansing agents or surfactants.

Natural shampoos

Many products contain natural substances derived from therapeutic plants and herbs. These are only considered to have a specific effect if they account for more than 5 per cent of the total. The percentage for essential oils is much lower — from 0.5 to 2.5 per cent, depending on the oil. If a product does not state the precise type and quantity of ingredients, you can assume that they were added purely for aesthetic appeal.

Conditioners

Conditioners are designed to restore the balance of natural oils after shampooing. Most commercial brands, although superficially effective, do little

Coconut oil is an excellent hair conditioner.

Vegetable oils include wheat germ and almond.

more than form an oily residue that 'sits' on the hair. Natural ingredients tend to be more biologically compatible with the hair. They leave your hair smooth and manageable, and also improve the texture.

Vegetable oils make effective conditioners. Any of the following are suitable: sesame, jojoba, coconut, sweet almond, apricot kernel or linseed; wheat germ works but smells less pleasant than the others.

- To help stimulate hair growth, add two drops of rosemary essential oil to the base oil.
- For an itchy scalp or dandruff, add a couple of drops of tea-tree oil to the base oil.

Wash your hair in the shower or over the sink, but apply a conditioning treatment (see page 96) while bathing for maximum benefit, because the warm atmosphere allows the ingredients to be absorbed more easily. Follow a conditioner of any kind with a natural hair rinse (see page 96) to enhance colour and shine.

pH Balance

The symbol pH indicates degrees of acidity or alkalinity: pH 7, the value for distilled water, is neutral; pH values 0–7 indicate acidity and 7–14 indicate alkalinity. Hair, like skin, has a pH of 4.5–5.5. Products that are too alkaline (the richer, 'thickening' shampoos, for example), or too acidic (mainly conditioners, cream rinses, and hair masks), can disturb this natural balance. Also, using a shampoo and conditioner with different pH balances can throw hair out of sync.

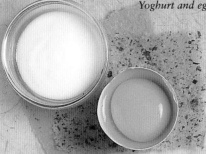

Yoghurt and egg yolk.

Yoghurt Conditioner
(for fine and flyaway hair)
YOU WILL NEED

6 tbsp (90ml/3fl oz) natural yoghurt

1 egg yolk (broken yolk with membrane removed)

Plastic shower cap

Towel, warmed

1 Blend the yoghurt and egg yolk together to a smooth paste.
2 Shampoo and rinse hair.
3 Towel dry and apply the mixture. Massage evenly into the hair.
4 Cover with a plastic shower cap to prevent staining, and wrap in a towel which has been warmed over a radiator — not over an open-flame fire or gas appliance.
5 Leave for 10–15 minutes. Rinse your hair thoroughly in lukewarm water.
6 Give hair a final rinse in cold water.

Olive Oil Conditioner
(for normal and dry/damaged hair)
YOU WILL NEED

2–3 tbsp (45ml/1½fl oz) warm olive oil

Warm towel

1 Saturate your hair with the warm olive oil. Wrap it in a warm towel and leave for 20 minutes. For extra benefits, give yourself a head massage (see box, page 19) while your hair is covered with oil.
2 Rinse with cold water, then shampoo. (Warm the oil in a container placed in a pan of hot water.)

Avocado Conditioner
(for dry and brittle hair)
YOU WILL NEED

2–3 ripe avocados (size according to amount of hair)

2 tsp (5ml/⅛fl oz) avocado oil

Plastic shower cap

Warm towel

1 Use a fork or blender to mash the avocados into enough pulp to cover your hair.
2 Add the avocado oil to form a paste.
3 Massage the mixture into your hair, concentrating on the ends.
4 Cover with a shower cap, and wrap in a warm towel. Leave for 15–20 minutes.
5 Rinse in lukewarm water.

Hair Rinses

Rinses help to remove traces of conditioner. They improve colour and leave your hair shiny and smooth.

Lemon Rinse (for oily hair)
Squeeze the juice from 3–4 lemons and add to a bowl of cold water. Use a jug to pour the solution over your hair. If your hair is long, swish it in the liquid. Rinse as usual.

Vinegar Rinse (for normal to greasy hair)
Add 1¼ cups (300ml/½pt) of vinegar to a bowl of cold water and rinse your hair in it. Give a final rinse in clear cold water.

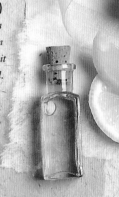

Lemons.

Herbal Tea Rinse (to enhance fair/ blonde hair)
Infuse 2–3 tea bags of camomile or calendula (marigold) in boiling water. Leave to cool, and rinse hair. Give a final rinse in cold water.

Herbal tea bag.

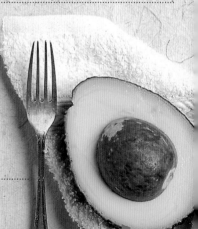

Ingredients

Throughout this book the author has recommended the use of many natural ingredients, either on their own or mixed with others. Pregnant women or nursing mothers, the very young or old, and people on medication should not use herbal remedies without a doctor's approval. For specific health problems, consult your doctor for guidance.

In this section we give helpful information about the ingredients and their uses.

Plants

The following ingredients can be used to make your own natural therapeutic remedies.

Aloe vera

A cactus-like evergreen plant. Applied externally, by placing a slice of leaf or some gel directly onto the skin. It is extremely soothing, and can help heal skin allergies and irritations. It is particularly effective for treating minor skin burns and sunburn.

Avocado (far left) is a natural and excellent hair conditioner. Aloe vera gel (below) is a perfect skin-soother.

Angelica (*Angelica archangelica*)

The leaves can be made into an infusion to stimulate circulation and ease respiratory problems. Good for colds and flu.
Caution Anyone at risk from heart disease should avoid recipes containing this herb.

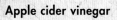
Apple and cider.

Apple cider vinegar

Has a pH balance that is naturally compatible with that of the skin and hair, so it helps to regulate the skin's pH balance. It also contains malic acid, a fruit acid which helps to remove dead skin cells. Can be added directly to the bath or used with cold water for rinsing your hair.

Arnica

Most frequently available as a tincture made up from the herb *Arnica montana*, it is excellent for bruises and aching muscles.

Caution Internal use is toxic. External use may cause a serious allergic reaction in some people.

Azuki beans

These pale pink, silky beans were first used in Japan. They are roasted to remove excess moisture and utilised to exfoliate and cleanse the skin.

Bran

The fibrous part of wheat. Add to the bath for its skin-smoothing properties, or use as an exfoliator.

Calendula (*Calendula officinalis*)

Used to soothe skin complaints, Calendula (pot marigold) has antiviral, antibacterial and anti-inflammatory properties. It can be the ingredient of a delicate moisturiser. Buy it as a tincture or a cream, or infuse some flowers to make a bath potion.
Caution Avoid during pregnancy.

Calendula (marigold)

Camomile (*Anthemis nobilis* or *Chamaemelum nobile*)

Camomile has skin-soothing properties and is generally calming. It is also antispasmodic; an infusion of these flowers added to the bath can help with cramps and spasms.

Chickweed (*Stellaria media*)

This common weed can be made (using flower heads and/or leaves) into a poultice, or brewed as a tea and added to the bath. It helps to relieve skin itching and inflammation caused by conditions such as eczema, allergies and rashes.

Echinacea augustifolia

Considered to be an antimicrobial herb — a natural antibiotic. It helps to strengthen the immune system and fight infection. Usually available in capsules or tablets to be taken orally, but you can buy echinacea as a root, brew it into a herbal decoction and apply it to septic sores and cuts. **Caution** Not recommended for pregnant women, nursing mothers, diabetics, or children under two. It should not be used by people suffering from severe illnesses such as multiple sclerosis, tuberculosis and all auto-immune diseases.

Fennel (*Foeniculum vulgare*)

Fennel seeds are rich in oils, which have an antispasmodic effect. Chewing fennel seeds also aids digestion. **Caution** Do not use for more than two weeks without medical supervision. Avoid if pregnant.

Echinacea flower and camomile heads.

Flaxseed (*Linum usitatissimum*)

Has emollient properties and soothes the mucous membrane, so is beneficial for chest infections and to relieve skin problems, such as shingles, boils and psoriasis. Make an infusion from the dried herb seed to apply as a poultice, or add to the bath. **Caution** Not to be taken internally in cases of intestinal obstruction.

Ginger (*Zingiber officinale*)

The root can be used fresh to make a warming decoction. Ginger is stimulating and helps to improve circulation and digestion. It is also good for aches and muscular pains. **Caution** Use during pregnancy should be supervised by a doctor. Overdose may cause cardiac arrhythmia and depress the central nervous system.

Honey

The sweet syrup made by bees has always been renowned for its natural antiseptic and immunity-boosting qualities. As a cosmetic, it moisturises the skin and a few spoonfuls added to your bath make your skin soft. Can also be added to other moisturisers.

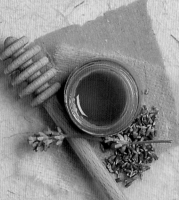

Honey and lavender.

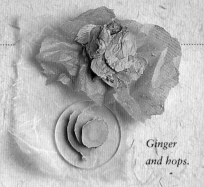

Ginger and hops.

Hops (*Humulus lupulus*)

These are classified as hypnotic herbs because of their sedative action. Made into an infusion and added to the bath, hops are useful for inducing feelings of deep relaxation and encouraging sleep. **Caution** May cause diarrhoea, stomach ache, or contact dermatitis in some people.

Lavender (*Lavandula spica* and *L. vera*)

A multipurpose herb that is healing and calming both mentally and to the skin. It helps balance the nervous system and possesses natural antiseptic and anti-inflammatory qualities.

Lemon balm (*Melissa officinalis*)

These fresh, lemon-scented leaves have an uplifting effect on the psyche and help relieve tension. Their anti-inflammatory properties soothe the skin. **Caution** Consult your doctor before use if you are suffering from thyroid-related problems.

Lime blossom (*Tilia americana*)

These flowers are soothing mentally and physically. Lime blossom helps to lower high blood pressure, and an infusion added to the bath encourages relaxation. An infusion made from lime flowers has a softening effect on the skin.
Caution Excessive use may cause cardiac toxicity.

Marsh mallow (*Althaea officinalis*)

A skin-soothing herb which can be used in a poultice to help heal wounds and draw out impurities. The whole plant can be used and the herb is often incorporated in soaps and moisturisers for its complexion-purifying properties.

Mint

The mint family includes peppermint (*Mentha piperita*) and spearmint (*Mentha spicata*). Mint has antispasmodic properties and is mentally uplifting. Mint tea makes an excellent digestive aid.

Mint.

Mustard

Black mustard (*Brassica nigra*) is used to make a warm poultice which is effective in relieving muscular and rheumatic pain.
Caution Prolonged external use can result in skin and nerve damage and should not exceed two weeks.

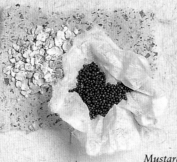

Mustard seeds and oats.

Oats

Oatmeal is a skin-softening agent and exfoliator. Especially good for sensitive skins. Make your own oatmeal pack (mix flakes with warm water, milk or yoghurt). Apply directly to the skin.

Passion flower (*Passiflora incarnata*)

A soothing herb, which helps to calm the nervous system and induce sleep. Use an infusion of the leaves in the bath.
Caution To be avoided by pregnant women.

Pine needle extract

Usually derived from the Scots or the Swiss pine tree, either as a powder or an oil. Stimulating and warming. Helps relieve muscular aches and pains. Has an invigorating effect on the psyche.
Caution Avoid during pregnancy. Can be toxic, especially in children.

Rice bran

Has skin-softening properties and makes an effective and gentle exfoliant.

Rose

The fruits, berries and petals of the rose bush can be made into an infusion that helps to calm and soothe the skin. Try adding some rose petals to your bathwater. Rosewater, a by-product from the steam distillation of rose essential oil, has anti-inflammatory properties when applied to an irritated or reddish complexion.

Passion flower blossom.

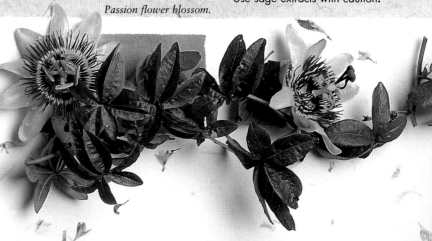

Rosemary (*Rosmarinus officinalis*)

This herb is renowned for its antiseptic and stimulating properties. An infusion of leaves added to the bath helps ease muscular aches and promotes better circulation. Used on the scalp, it may improve hair growth and eliminate dandruff.
Caution Do not use internally during pregnancy. Can cause dermatitis in some people.

Sage (*Salvia officinalis*)

From the north Mediterranean area. This herb has natural antibiotic properties. An infusion of leaves used as a mouthwash helps sore throats.
Caution Pregnant women and nursing mothers should avoid the herb altogether. Do not ingest sage oil, or apply it externally. Use sage extracts with caution.

Thyme (*Thymus vulgaris*)

The leaves possess antiviral, antifungal and antibacterial properties. Thyme helps with urinary, skin and other infections. It is warming and stimulating.

Caution Medicinal amounts are contra-indicated in cases of enterocolitis and cardiac insufficiency, and should not be taken by pregnant women, nursing mothers, or those with an overactive thyroid.

Valerian (*Valeriana officinalis*)

A hypnotic, naturally sedative herb, renowned for its sleep-inducing properties. Can be taken orally as a tincture, or as an infusion added to the bath.

Walnut

The dried leaves from the English walnut tree (*Juglans regia*) can be brewed to make an infusion. Use as a hair rinse to darken the hair.

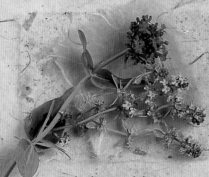

Red valerian and thyme.

Wheat germ

Has similar properties to oatmeal. Soothes the skin and makes a good natural exfoliant.

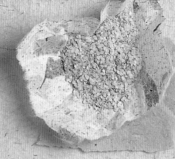

Wheat germ.

Witch hazel (*Hamamelis virginiana*)

Witch hazel leaves possess anti-inflammatory and astringent properties. An infusion of these helps to relieve itchy skin. Witch hazel is most often available as a lotion, which makes a good natural toner for the complexion.

Yarrow (*Achillea millefolium*)

This is an astringent, styptic diaphoretic herb (promotes sweating). An infusion of the leaves is detoxifying and will help you to sweat out a cold. It also improves circulation.

Caution Should not be ingested by pregnant women.

Oils

Essential oils are too highly concentrated to be used directly on the skin so always dilute them first in a carrier oil.

ESSENTIAL OILS

This list of the most popular oils describes their main properties. Choose suitable ones to use in the bath, to add to massage oil, or to use in an oil burner.

Caution *Do not ingest essential oils.*

Bergamot oil (*Citrus bergamia*)

A light greeny-yellow liquid, extracted from the peel of the fruit. Has a fresh citrus scent.

Main properties uplifting, reviving, balancing.
Used for anxiety, depression, colds, infections, skin problems.
Caution Do not take bergamot essential oil internally.

Cardamom oil (*Elettaria cardamomum*)

Spicy, oriental-scented oil extracted from cardamom seeds (found in India).

Main properties antispasmodic, antiseptic, aphrodisiac.
Used for mental fatigue, flatulence, indigestion.
Caution Do not take cardamon essential oil internally.

How to Use Essential Oils

Essential oils achieve their effects chiefly through inhalation and absorption through the skin when used in the following ways:
- *Massage: 2–3 drops diluted in a carrier oil and warmed in the hands.*
- *Compress: 1–2 drops on a pad or handkerchief.*
- *Inhalation: 8–12 drops in a bowl of warm water.*
- *Bath: 3–6 drops in a carrier oil diluted in the water. This is one of the best methods, because you absorb the oils simultaneously through the olfactory nerves and the skin.*

Essential oils are highly volatile and penetrate the skin through their unique molecular structure, which enables the vapours to pass through by diffusion. Once inside the skin, they pass into the bloodstream, which carries them to the internal organs. Inhaled essential oils travel through the olfactory nerves to the brain and are also diffused into the bloodstream via the respiratory system.

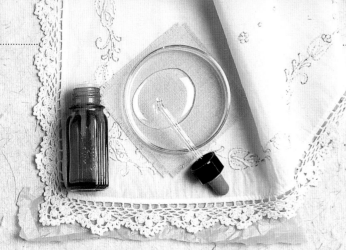

Camomile oil.

Camomile oil (German: *Matricaria recutita*)

A herby, warm oil derived from camomile flowers.

Main properties calming, sedative, antispasmodic.

Used for allergies, pimples, inflammation, rashes, stomach cramps, anxiety, insomnia and headaches.

Caution Do not take the essential oil internally except under professional supervision.

Camomile oil (Roman: *Chamaemelum nobile*)

Distinctive smelling oil extracted from the heads of the flowers.

Main properties calming, sedative, relaxing, antispasmodic, digestive.

Used for allergies, inflammation, rashes, stomach cramps, anxiety, insomnia and headaches.

Caution Do not take the essential oil internally except under professional supervision.

Cedarwood oil (*Cedrus atlantica*)

A sweet, woody, amber-coloured oil derived from the wood of the Atlas cedar tree.

Main property reviving.

Used for acne, problem skin, congestion, coughs and catarrh.

Caution Do not take the essential oil internally except under professional supervision. Do not use while pregnant.

Clary sage oil (*Salvia sclarea*)

A richly scented musky oil derived from the leaves of the clary sage plant.

Main properties sedative, aphrodisiac.

Used for greasy skin, depression, low libido, high blood pressure.

Caution Do not take the essential oil internally except under professional supervision. Do not use while pregnant.

Cypress oil (*Cupressus sempervirens*)

A woody oil extracted from the leaves and twigs of the Italian cypress.

Main properties soothing, refreshing, astringent.

Used for greasy skin, water retention, painful menstruation.

Caution Do not take the essential oil internally except under professional supervision.

Eucalyptus oil (*Eucalyptus globulus*)

A fresh-scented oil derived from the twigs and leaves of blue-gum eucalyptus trees.

Main properties expectorant, antiviral, antiseptic, analgesic.

Used for asthma, bronchitis, catarrh, colds, flu, respiratory problems and viral infections.

Caution Do not take the essential oil internally except under professional supervision.

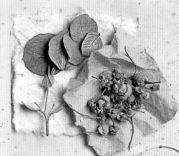

Grapefruit rind, eucalyptus and geranium.

Frankincense oil (*Buswellia thurifera*)

A balsamic, woody oil extracted from bark resin (found in the Middle East, Somalia, China and Ethiopia).

Main properties purifying, calming, revitalising, restorative.

Used for dry skin, blemishes, scars and to relieve nervous tension. Frankincense is also burned as an incense to induce calmness for prayer and meditation.

Geranium oil (*Pelargonium graveolens*)

Fresh-smelling oil extracted from the leaves and flowers of the rose geranium plant.

Main properties anti-inflammatory, uplifting, balancing.

Used for dry skins, blemishes, nervous tension, cellulite.

Grapefruit oil (*Citrus paradisi*)

A bitter, citrus-scented oil extracted from the rind.

Main properties refreshing, cleansing, energising.

Used for cellulite and to boost energy levels.

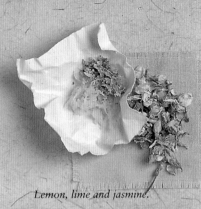

Lemon, lime and jasmine.

Jasmine oil (*Jasminum officinale*)

An intoxicating, exotic, warm-scented oil extracted from jasmine flowers (found in France, Egypt, Morocco, Algeria and China). After rose, this is the most expensive oil to produce.
Main properties balancing, warming, aphrodisiac, euphoric.
Used for sensitive skin, loss of libido, stress.

Lavender oil (*Lavandula spica* and *L. vera*)

A light, floral oil extracted from lavender flowers.
Main properties sedative, calming, purifying, antiseptic, stimulating.
Used for skin problems, pimples, acne, colds, bronchitis, muscular aches and pains, insomnia, nervous tension.

Lemon oil (*Citrus limon*)

Refreshing, fruit-scented oil extracted from the rind.
Main properties antiseptic, mentally stimulating, purifying.
Used for boils, pimples, insect bites, throat infections, catarrh.

Lime oil (*Citrus aurantifolia*)

Fresh, sharp citrus-scented oil extracted from the rind.
Main properties refreshing, uplifting, antiseptic.
Used for acne, colds.

Mandarin oil (*Citrus reticulata*)

A sweet citrus oil extracted from the rind.
Main properties warming, soothing.
Used for nervous tension, problem skin.

Lavender.

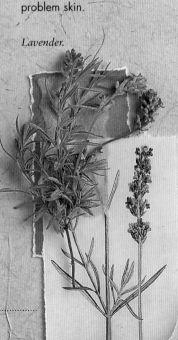

Neroli oil (*Citrus aurantium*)

Derived from orange blossom.
Main properties antiseptic, antispasmodic, aphrodisiac, antidepressant, uplifting.
Used for dry skins, stretch marks, blemishes, anxiety, depression, PMS.

Orange oil (sweet) (*Citrus sinensis*)

A fruity citrus oil extracted from the rind of an orange.
Main properties uplifting, tonic.
Used for greasy skin, to calm nervous tension.

Patchouli oil (*Pogostemon cablin*)

A musk-scented oil derived from the patchouli plant.
Main properties antidepressant, sedative, aphrodisiac, uplifting.
Used for greasy skin, relaxation, loss of libido.

Peppermint oil (*Mentha piperita*)

Fresh, mint-scented oil extracted from the whole plant.
Main properties anti-inflammatory, decongestant, refreshing, stimulating, uplifting.
Used for muscular pains, indigestion, colic, colds and flu, and to boost energy levels.
Caution Can irritate sensitive skin and cause dizziness; do not use when pregnant or if taking homeopathic remedies as mint has an antidote effect. Do not prescribe to children.

Rose oil (*Rosa damascena* and *Rosa maroc*)

A warm, floral oil extracted from the petals of the Bulgarian and the Moroccan rose. A pure 'rose absolut' is the most expensive oil to produce.
Main properties aphrodisiac, calming, uplifting, balancing.
Used for dry, mature skins, depression, frigidity, poor circulation.
Caution Avoid if pregnant.

Rosemary.

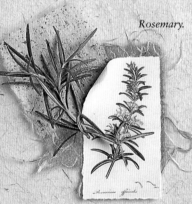

Rosemary oil (*Rosmarinus officinalis*)

Fresh, herby oil extracted from the leaves and flowers.
Main properties antiseptic, stimulating, antibacterial.
Used for skin problems, allergies, colds, flu, infections, muscle aches and pains.
Caution Avoid if pregnant.

Sandalwood oil
(*Santalum album*)

A dry, woody oil derived from the wood of the sandalwood tree grown in Indonesia and India.
Main properties antiseptic, antidepressant, aphrodisiac, balancing.
Used for acne, boils, pimples, depression, cramps.

Rose.

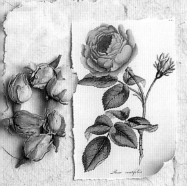

Tea-tree oil
(*Melaleuca alternifolia*)

A strong medicinal-smelling oil extracted from the leaves and twigs of the tea tree found in Australia and Tasmania.
Main properties antifungal, antiseptic, antibacterial.
Used for acne, insect bites, abscesses, boils, fungal infections, colds and flu.

Ylang-ylang oil
(*Cananga odorata*)

A sweet, exotic, sensual oil derived from ylang-ylang flowers found in the Philippines, Indonesia, and the Comoro Islands.
Main properties sedative, calming, aphrodisiac, soothing.
Used for skin irritations, loss of libido, depression, relaxation.

VEGETABLE AND CARRIER OILS

Carrier, or base, oils are derived from vegetables, seeds, nuts and plants. They have therapeutic properties in their own right, and can be used alone or mixed with a few drops of essential oil to improve the condition of your skin and hair. They are also good for massage. Each oil varies in texture: the lighter and more absorbent oils suit normal to oily skins; the thicker, richer oils are better for dry skins. They can be used to make soaps, conditioners and moisturisers.
Caution Avoid any nut-based oils (including almond and apricot kernel) if you have an allergy to nuts.

Almond oil (sweet)
(*Amygdalus communis*)

A pale, yellow oil derived from sweet almonds. Contains minerals, vitamins and proteins. Helps relieve itchy skin. Suitable for most skin types.

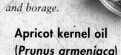

Apricot kernel and borage.

Apricot kernel oil
(*Prunus armeniaca*)

A pale, yellow oil derived from the kernel. This oil is considered to have natural anti-wrinkle properties. Apricot kernel oil makes a good general moisturiser. Suitable for all skin types.

Avocado oil
(*Persea americana*)

A dark green oil made from the fruit. Avocados are rich in vitamin A, lecithin, fatty acids and natural oils. Use avocado oil as a moisturiser, facepack or hair conditioner. Suitable for dry, mature skins.

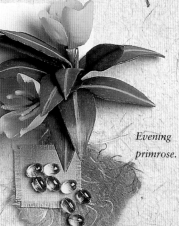

Evening primrose.

Borage oil
(*Borago officinalis*)

A yellow oil made from borage seeds. Contains gamma linoleic acid, vitamins and minerals. Use blended with other carrier oils. Suitable for all skin types.

Coconut oil (*Cocus nucifera*)

Derived from the dried flesh of the coconut. Highly moisturising for skin and hair. Often used in shampoos and soaps. Rich in vitamins and minerals. Suitable for dry skin.

Corn oil (*Zea mays*)

A pale, yellow oil rich in proteins, vitamins and minerals. Can be used as a soothing base oil on all skin types.

Evening primrose oil
(*Oenothera biennis*)

A pale, yellow oil made from evening primrose flowers. Rich in gamma linoleic acid, vitamins and minerals. Helps relieve symptoms of eczema and psoriasis. Suitable for dry, sensitive and mature skins.

Wakame.

Grapeseed and sesame seed in safflower oil.

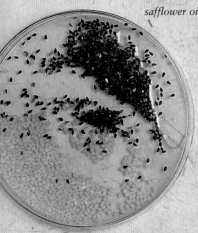

Grapeseed oil (*Vinifera* vars.)

A light, colourless oil made from grapeseeds. Contains vitamins and minerals. Is emollient and not too greasy. Suitable for all skin types.

Jojoba oil (*Simmondsia californica*)

A yellow oil made from the jojoba bean. Slightly waxy in texture. Contains proteins and minerals. Helps soothe eczema and psoriasis. Highly moisturising, and especially good for sensitive, dry skins.

Olive oil (*Olea europaea*)

A rich, greenish oil made from olives. Rich in vitamins and minerals. Good for dry skins.

Safflower oil (*Carthamus tinctorius*)

A pale, yellow oil extracted from the thistle-like safflower plant. Very moisturising and suitable for all skin types.

Sesame oil (*Sesamum indicum*)

A dark, yellow oil derived from the sesame plant. Rich in vitamins, minerals, lecithin and proteins. A popular oil in very hot countries because it is slow to go rancid. It also offers some protection from the sun's rays so it is often used in suntan lotions. Suitable for all skin types.

Wheat germ oil (*Triticum* vars.)

An orange-coloured oil, rich in vitamins, minerals and proteins. Helps eczema and psoriasis symptoms. Good for dry and dehydrated skins.

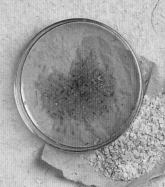

Wheat germ oil.

Minerals

Minerals constitute only 4–5 per cent of your body weight, yet they and other trace elements are essential for good health.

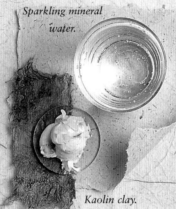

Sparkling mineral water.

Kaolin clay.

Minerals are necessary for a wide range of functions, including the formation and maintenance of soft tissue, muscle, and blood and nerve cells. They also help to keep the heart and brain healthy. Minerals act as catalysts for many biochemical reactions; nerve transmission, the utilisation of nutrients from foods, digestion, and proper hormone function. They work to maintain correct water balance and stabilise levels of acidity and alkalinity within the system. Deficiencies can lead to many problems affecting general health.

The body cannot make minerals and must obtain them through diet and water. Food derived from unpolluted land, bottled spa water, bathing in spa water and taking supplements are the best ways to ensure that you are meeting your mineral requirements. Mud, clay and seaweed therapeutic treatments are another excellent means of enabling minerals and trace elements to be absorbed by the body (see pages 40–7). Right are details of some of the most important minerals that your body needs.

Mineral water

Bottled spa waters are also a source of mineral salts. The most common ingredients are bicarbonates, sulphates, nitrates, chlorides and calcium. To find the most suitable water for you, consult the label on the bottle, which gives an analysis of the mineral salts it contains.

Kelp.

Kombu.

Bladderwrack.

Which Seaweed?

Seaweeds vary according to area of origin. These are some of the varieties most frequently used in thalassotherapy preparations.

Type of seaweed	Description	Properties
Bladderwrack (Fucus vesiculosus)	A brown algae from the Atlantic Ocean and English Channel.	Softening, anti-inflammatory, rebalancing and detoxifying.
Laminaria digitata	A brown algae found in the Atlantic Ocean and English Channel.	Rich in iodine and mineral salts. Stimulates the metabolism, fosters efficient functioning, diuretic.
Christe marine (also named Perce Pierre)	A sea plant found off the coast of Brittany, France.	Rich in iodine and vitamin C. Diuretic and detoxifying.
Wakame	A Japanese sea plant.	Rich in kelp and mineral salts. Stimulates circulation, softens skin and improves skin tone.
Kombu	A Japanese sea plant.	Rich in vitamins and mineral salts. Stimulates circulation, improves skin tone, detoxifying.

BENEFITS OF MINERALS

These minerals are commonly found in natural springs:

- **Sulphur** Essential for the formation of red blood cells.
- **Iron** Necessary for the formation of the blood's haemoglobin and myoglobin.
- **Silica** Helps to regulate blood pressure.
- **Calcium** Required for healthy bones and teeth.
- **Sodium** Ensures the correct balance of water in cells.
- **Zinc** Essential for rebuilding the body's cells.
- **Potassium** Balances cell metabolism.

MINERAL THERAPY

You can enjoy the benefits of a mineral bath at home.

- Silicon dioxide (fine sand) can be used as a coarse exfoliator for very rough areas, such as the soles of the feet.
- To exfoliate the skin or remove dry, rough patches, make a salt paste by mixing 115g (4oz) coarse sea salt with jojoba or almond oil. Use a soft body brush or mitt on areas such as knees and elbows.
- To cleanse the skin, open pores, and help skin irritation, add 225g (8oz) baking soda to the bath.
- To induce perspiration, get rid of toxins, and relax the muscles, add 225–450g (8–16oz) of Epsom salts to a warm bath and soak for 20 minutes.

Sea salt.

Baking soda.

Epsom salts.

Silicon dioxide (sand).

Caution Do not use if you suffer from diabetes, high blood pressure, or heart problems.

A range of minerals, from sea salt to baking soda, can be therapeutic.

WATER ELIXIRS

We are surrounded by crystals. They form 85 per cent of the earth's rocks and are even present inside our bodies. Crystals make up mountains and ocean floors. But what exactly are they? Crystalline particles are made up of solidified minerals and ever since they were first discovered, people have always been fascinated by their many various shapes and colours. Crystals are one of the easiest ingredients to use in a water elixir. They have long been revered for their healing properties, which are believed to be based on the energy 'vibrations' they emit. These stem in part from their specific colour. Each colour has a different 'vibration' that can be measured in wavelengths of light. The theory is that when you hold or wear a crystal, its natural energy field influences the energies of your body. You can capture the crystal's energies in a water elixir.

Sea salt.

Gem Elixir

YOU WILL NEED

Selected crystal(s)

2 tbsp (30ml) sea salt

5 cups (1.2 litres) spring water

Glass dropper bottle (sterilised)

Glass jar

1 Charge the crystal by leaving it to soak in a salt-water solution.
2 Pat the crystal dry, and leave it in a sunny place outdoors for 3–4 hours.
3 Put the crystal in the glass jar and fill the jar with spring water. Cover the jar and leave for 24 hours on a natural surface. Transfer into the glass dropper bottle and store in a cool place.
4 Use the elixir to create a spray mist. Alternatively, add 5–10 drops to your bath. Do not keep for longer than three days.

Aquamarine.

Clear quartz.

Topaz.

Crystal properties

Crystals are reputed to aid mental as well as physical well-being. When making an elixir choose the appropriate gem:

Gem	Properties
Aquamarine	Calming, detoxifying. Inspires creativity and self-expression.
Citrine	Raises self-esteem; boosts confidence.
Fluorite	Reduces anxiety and frustration.
Jasper	Calms and soothes the psyche.
Lapis lazuli	Increases self-confidence; promotes self-expression.
Malachite	Cleansing and rebalancing.
Opal	Promotes an open mind, receptive to new ideas.
Clear quartz	Boosts mental activity. Calming.
Rose quartz	Soothes. Inspires optimism.
Sapphire	Improves intuition. Promotes psychic clarity.
Topaz	Helps to deal with anger, jealousy, and depression.
Turquoise	Balancing. Promotes general healing. Offers protection.

Spas

The last ten years have seen a change in attitude towards holidays. Studies of skin cancer and premature ageing have cancelled, for many, the attractions of sunbathing for hours on a sun-soaked beach. A greater awareness of personal fitness has reduced the appeal of lengthy lounging and over-indulgence. With stress levels constantly rising, many holidaymakers now want a short or long break that gives them the opportunity to unwind and generally rebalance before stepping back into the rat race. What better place to do it than a health resort or spa?

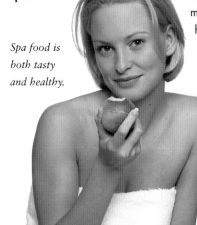

Spa food is both tasty and healthy.

What to Expect at a Spa

There was a time when the word 'spa' conjured up twin images. Spas were perceived as strict places, where you were woken with a cold shower and ate lettuce leaves all day. They were likely to be frequented by the rich and famous when they needed to shed a pound or two.

Today both stereotypes are out-of-date. With the demand for health and fitness holidays, the spa has undergone a total makeover. There are now hundreds of spas to choose from, according to preference, in almost every part of the world. They are often an additional attraction in hotels and resorts that offer a variety of recreation and entertainment, so that you can incorporate healthy spa activities into a regular holiday. Even traditional spas have

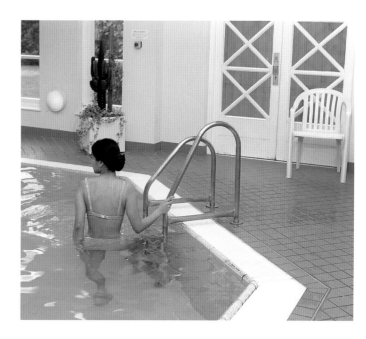

moved with the times. Most now offer typical water therapy regimes within a luxurious environment that includes restaurants, bars, entertainment and sports facilities. Increased demand has brought prices down, and it is possible for everyone to find a spa holiday to suit their budget. Spas are attracting people of all ages and walks of life, who want to promote their general well-being, and not just to treat a specific health condition.

Water therapy, from swimming for enjoyment to healing treatments, is a key feature of spa resorts.

Spa Therapies

Although treatments vary according to the spa's location, the basic therapies normally comprise different massages and diets, customised exercise programmes and beauty care, including facials and manicures. Most spas offer alternative treatments, such as reflexology and aromatherapy. There may

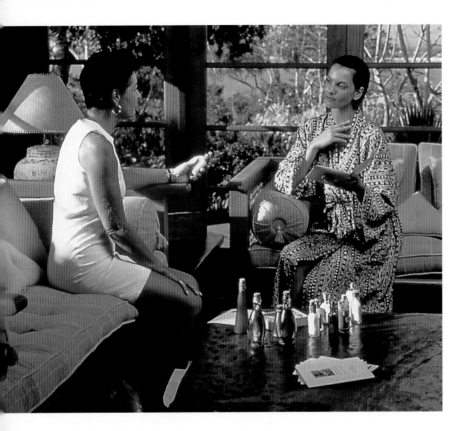

A stay at a spa begins with a consultation like this one at a resort in Bali, to assess your personal needs.

be talks on complementary therapies, nutrition and other topics relating to health and fitness. A spa generally has sports and fitness facilities, such as a gym, swimming pool and tennis courts, and offers optional organised walks, hikes, cycling and other activities. Doctors, nutritionists, and fitness instructors are on hand to give you a personal health consultation before you begin your programme.

Which Spa?

Like any other holiday or weekend destination, spas cater for a variety of tastes and needs. So before you choose, check out exactly what's on offer.

The Classic Spa The traditional spa is usually self-contained. Typical examples are The Palms at Palm Springs and Canyon Ranch, in the US, and Champneys Health Resort in the UK. Such spas are usually at the top end of the scale and offer fairly intense regimes amid luxurious surroundings. The emphasis is on a healthy diet, exercise, and personal choice from all of the therapeutic and beauty treatments that you could wish to find in a spa. Restrictions on smoking and alcohol consumption tend to be stricter here than in many other spas. Classic spas are normally located in exquisite, off-the-beaten-track surroundings, and privacy is paramount.

Luxury Spas These include exclusive resorts, such as Cal-a-Vie in California or the Doral Saturnia in Miami. They include all of the luxuries you could dream of, and pride themselves on their superb cuisine. They are also set in fabulous locations. The guest list is smaller than in many other spas, and there is plenty of privacy. These are a good choice for celebrating a special occasion, or if you just want to be utterly pampered.

Weight-loss Spas Centres such as the Bermuda Inn Fitness Resort, California, offer exclusive weight-loss programmes, based on healthy, sensible eating plans. The days of starvation diets are over. What these spas do is help you to re-educate your approach to how you eat. They aim to improve your nutritional habits and motivation, so when you leave, slimmer and fitter, you will be set to stay that way. You will be armed with a new attitude to eating, which should prevent you from falling back into unhealthy patterns.

New Age Spas Although most spas today offer a comprehensive range of alternative treatments, such as reflexology, shiatsu, aromatherapy massage and stress-reduction programmes, some spas specialise in such therapies. At a new age spa, such as the Maharishi Ayur-Veda Health Centre, in

Massachusetts, the focus is on rebalancing the body and mind with an array of complementary treatments. These spas take a holistic approach to the individual, and a stay at one of them can have powerful life-changing effects.

Resort or Hotel-based Spas
Visiting a spa attached to the hotel, or within the resort where you are staying, is a good way of discovering whether or not a spa is for you. You can dip into the spa facilities as you please while enjoying a more conventional holiday at the same time. This is a popular choice, because it combines favourite holiday attractions, such as restaurants and nightclubs, with a healthy backup — so that people can enjoy the best of both worlds.

Thalassotherapy Centres and Mineral Spas
These are renowned for their therapeutic water treatments, and are located close to naturally occurring hot springs or thermal water sources — or, in the case of thalassotherapy, near the sea. They are an excellent choice if you suffer from a specific condition, such as rheumatism or skin problems, because they offer a host of treatments to alleviate, or even cure, particular ailments — and their success rate is high. However, anyone can enjoy these beautiful, natural healing places, and you are sure to come back feeling rejuvenated.

What to Take to a Spa
Ideally, very little. The beauty of staying at a spa is that no matter how exclusive it is, you can lounge all day long in a fluffy, towelling robe and swimsuit, or casual sports clothes. Check, though, on the dress code for the evenings. At many spas you can wear casual clothes throughout, but in a hotel or at a luxury spa, you need to dress up for dinner. Check also on local weather; if the spa is located in a hot climate, be sure to pack enough swimwear, shorts and T-shirts. Take warm sweaters, jackets, and walking boots if you plan to do a lot of hiking in colder places. Most spas have a shop that carries basic items, including personal care products and clothes — although these tend to be expensive, they are convenient if you forget anything.

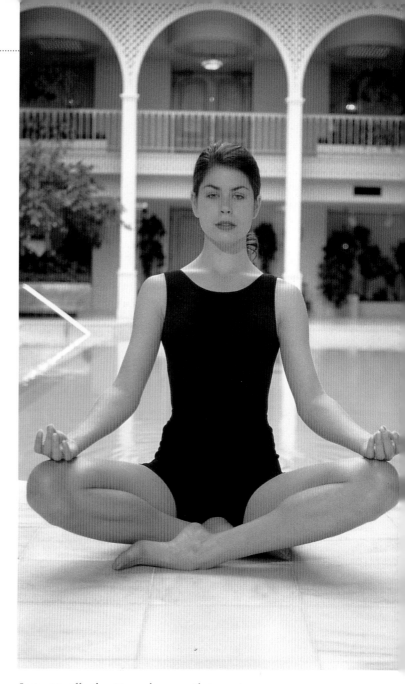

Some spas offer therapies such as yoga that exercise the mind and spirit as well as the body.

A One-day Stay at a Spa

Most spas offer day packages. These are useful if you want to pamper yourself and haven't time for an extended visit. You might think that one day isn't long enough to experience the full benefits. It is. By the end of your visit you will be surprised how wonderfully rejuvenating a single day of total relaxation can be.

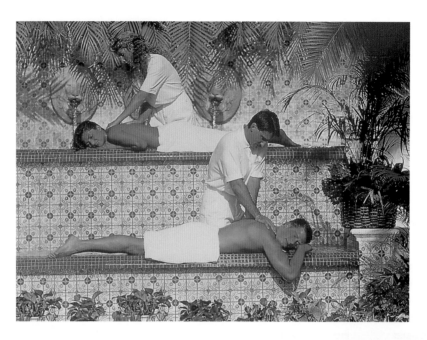

A relaxing massage at a spa in Florida. Most of the resorts offer an array of soothing, reviving, and healing massages.

Facial toning procedures can smooth your skin and enhance your appearance in the most relaxing way.

Choose a spa and check if they offer any special deals. Many do this for occasions such as Mother's Day, Valentine's Day, or as a short spring or autumn break. A package like this is more affordable, and much less expensive than booking all of the different treatments from separate sources.

What Happens?

A typical day's package is usually all-inclusive, which means you pay a fixed price and can choose from a number of options. Breakfast, lunch and afternoon refreshments are included. Your day will probably begin at around 9 am and end at around 6 pm.

You can enjoy going on your own, but many people like to take a friend or partner. When you arrive, you will be offered a light breakfast and then asked to choose from a selection of treatments and activities. Locker rooms, complete with showers, are available for changing out of your clothes and into a robe provided for you. You may also be given a pair of spa slippers. Take a swimsuit with you.

You will first be given a general fitness assessment and asked to fill out a questionnaire. Be sure to point out if you have any major or minor medical condition, such as high blood pressure, diabetes, allergies, or respiratory problems, or if you are pregnant. Mention any medication you are taking. This is important to avoid the possibility of an adverse reaction to one of the treatments — the sauna or steam room, for example.

After your individual consultation, a schedule will be devised for you, based on your preferred activities. Most day packages cover about three treatments. If you want — and have time for — additional therapies, you will need to pay extra.

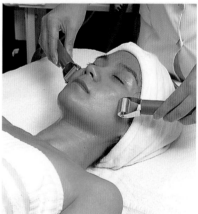

Treatments usually include a choice of massage, such as aromatherapy, Swedish massage, or shiatsu, which lasts about an hour. You will also be offered a choice of

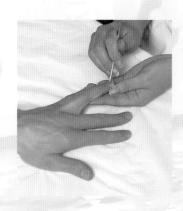

Try to pick up home-care tips when you have a manicure.

beauty treatments, such as a facial or manicure (sometimes both). A third option might be a hydrotherapy treatment, such as a water massage bath, using massage shower jets, or a body wrap with mud or seaweed. The range of treatments offered varies according to the spa.

The treatments are spread through the day; usually one before lunch, and two in the afternoon. If you plan to have a beauty treatment, leave it till last. After each session, drink plenty of the water provided, because some of the treatments are dehydrating. You should also rest for 15–20 minutes afterwards in one of the designated rooms. These contain 'loungers' on which you can just relax in your robe. This is important as you may initially feel lightheaded after certain therapies, such as a massage.

Throughout the rest of the day, the aim is to unwind. Lunch is usually a light buffet, with a choice of hot and cold nutritious food, followed by herbal tea. While you are at the spa you can try out the fitness and sports facilities between treatments — go for a swim, take a sauna, play some tennis. Take trainers or tennis shoes and some fitness clothes, if you plan to do any of these activities. There may also be exercise classes that you can attend during the day;

stretching, body conditioning or yoga, for example. Although it is tempting to cram in as much as possible, it is better to pace yourself. You will probably be more active than usual anyway. By the time you have a relaxing shower at the end of the day, you should be feeling thoroughly calm and refreshed.

Relaxing after a pampering session is one joy of a spa visit.

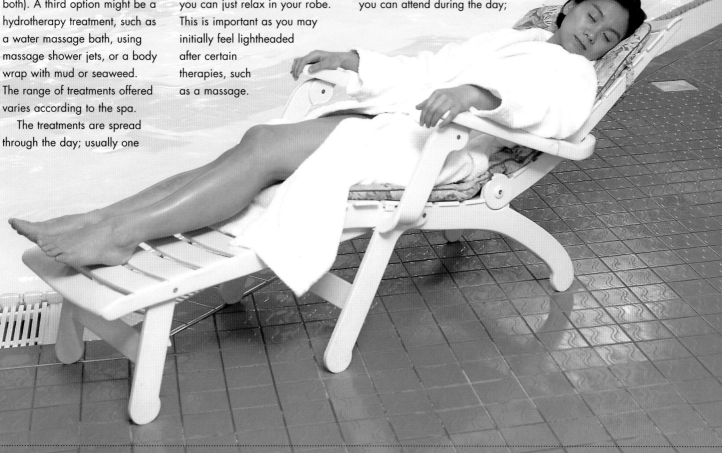

$\mathcal{P}$remier spas

This section of the book gives a selection of some of the best spas and health resorts in the world. Unfortunately, space does not allow for the choice of entries in this directory of 'Premier spas' to be entirely comprehensive — nor to give full descriptions of the facilities. Instead, it is intended as a reference for those spas that the author has personally chosen, either for their speciality treatments or for their diverse facilities, so that you, the reader, may find a spa you may regard as a haven, away from the everyday world, whether it be in your locality or at a favourite holiday spot.

NB: For British residents: dial 00 and then the country code before dialling the area codes and numbers outside the United Kingdom.

$\mathcal{N}$orth America

CANADA
The Pillar and Post Inn
Set near the Canadian banks of Niagara Falls, the Pillar and Post Inn is a charming refurbished canning factory filled with antiques, four-posters and fireside dining. The 100 Fountain Spa features state-of-the-art health facilities, a hot-spring pool and a solar-heated pool, plus a variety of massages, facials and bodywraps.
48 John Street, P.O. Box 1011, Niagara-on-the-Lake, Ontario, LOS IJO.
Tel: 1 800 361 6788

Auberge Parc Inn
Expect personal attention at this small but beautiful resort that caters for only 40 guests at a time. The European-style treatments of thalassotherapy, include sea-water baths, algae wrapping and therapeutic massage. Outdoors there is a nine-hole golf course, skiing, cycling and fishing.
C.P.40, Paspébiac, Québéc GOC 2KO.
Tel: 1 800 463 0890

Solace — The Spa at Banff Springs Hotel
Its philosophy is health through water and there are a variety of mineral and herb baths, facials, wraps and massages designed to help guests to relax thoroughly. Skiing and golf are available for the more energetic. Start the day with the cereal bar at the Solace Life Restaurant which features a mountain of healthy grains, fruit and nuts.
P.O. Box 960 or 405 Spray Street, Banff, Alberta, TDL OCO.
Tel: 1 800 404 1772

Mountain Trek Fitness Retreat & Health Spa
Mountain Trek combines pampering with three to six-hour hikes through some of the most spectacular scenery in North America. A perfect place to get away from it all, there are only 13 guests at a time. Log fires

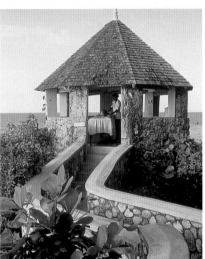

One of the luxurious facilities overlooking the Caribbean at Jamaica's Grand Sans Souci Lido, where recreation and health meet.

and a nearby hot spring help relax sore muscles at night, after a long, hard day.
Ainsworth Hot Springs, British Columbia.
Tel: 1 800 661 5161

JAMAICA
Royal Court Hotel and Natural Health Retreat, Montego Bay
Decorated in typically Jamaican style, the Royal Court Hotel offers a tranquil, private retreat. Treatments include yoga, bodywork, stress-management, a fully equipped gym, fitness classes, sauna, steam room

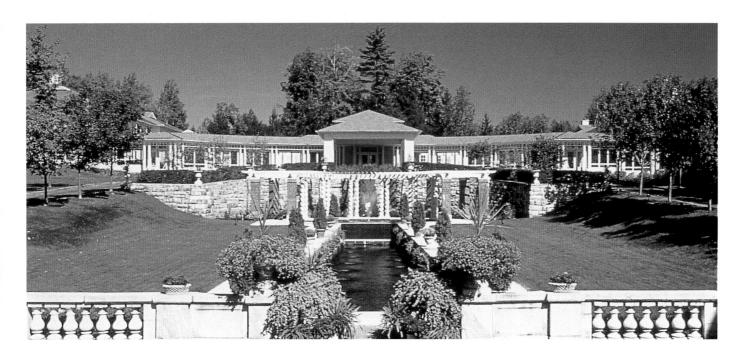

and beauty treatments. Food includes traditional Jamaican cuisine, with plenty of fresh tropical fruits.
Sewell Avenue, Montego Bay, St James, Jamaica, West Indies.
Tel: 1 876 952 4531

Sans Souci Lido, Ocho Rios

Provides an all-inclusive healthy holiday, where you can combine relaxation with a typical spa regime. There is an outdoor mineral-water pool that leaves the skin glowing. One of the best features is the gym, on the beach overlooking the sea. There are numerous fitness classes daily, including yoga

and body conditioning. Spa treatments comprise massages and thalassotherapy. There is also a beauty salon. A variety of restaurants serve Jamaican, Italian, international and light spa cuisine. The accommodation is exceptionally luxurious.
White River, Ocho Rios, St Ann, Jamaica, West Indies.
Tel: 1 876 994 1206–9

UNITED STATES
Arizona
Canyon Ranch

This world-renowned spa, in the heart of Arizona, offers an extensive list of health and fitness programmes. Spa

specialties include a pain-management programme, which is especially useful for arthritis sufferers, a stop smoking, and a postnatal programme. Alongside these is a variety of health and beauty regimes, including stretching and toning classes, aerobics, all kinds of fitness facilities, wraps, baths and beauty treatments.
8600 East Rockcliff Road, Tucson, AZ 85750.
Tel: 1 800 742 9000

California
Cal-a-Vie

In a canyon setting, amid acres of rolling hills dotted with pastel

The elegant splendour of the Canyon Ranch spa in Arizona houses a vast array of health, fitness, and beauty programmes, treatment and equipment.

cottages, Cal-a-Vie looks like a Mediterranean village. Superb facilities include hydrotherapy, thalassotherapy, plant extract massages and shiatsu, and exclusive skin treatments based on herbs and flowers grown on the premises. Excellent cuisine, ranging from luxury gourmet to spa menus.
2249 Somerset Road, Vista, CA 92084.
Tel: 1 760 945 2055

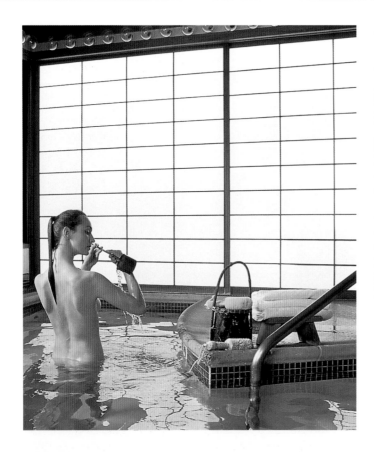

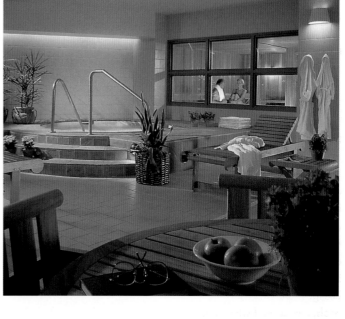

Attention to every detail of decor and landscaping makes the Golden Door Spa in California an authentic reflection of the East.

The Peaks at Telluride in the Rocky Mountains of Colorado has all the regular spa amenities, as well as mountain air and an impressive choice of sports.

Golden Door Spa

Designed to recreate an authentic Eastern style, Golden Door comprises soothing landscapes of ornamental and rock gardens, and bird sanctuaries. Every room has its own garden. In addition to a wide array of sports, fitness, health and beauty treatments, you can choose from more esoteric classes on life-enhancement techniques. The food is mainly nouvelle cuisine, utilising the exotic fruits that grow in the area.
PO Box 463077, Escondido, San Diego, CA 92046.
Tel: 1 760 744 5777

The Palms

Located at Palm Springs in the California desert, The Palms offers a comfortable, informal environment. The emphasis is on fitness and relaxation. You can choose to sign up for 5 km (3 mile) runs in the morning, and/or fitness classes of every description. There is a selection of beauty treatments. Food is classic spa style — light and healthy. There is also a 21-day Stop Smoking programme.
572 North Indian Canyon Drive, Palm Springs, CA 92262.
Tel: 1 760 325 1111

Marriott Desert Springs Resort and Spa

A European-style spa within the luxury Marriott Resort. Offers Turkish steam rooms, Finnish saunas, hot and cold plunge pools, whirlpools, aerobics studios, a fully equipped gym and an Olympic-sized swimming pool. There is a wide selection of health and beauty treatments, including aromatherapy, Swedish massage, herbal wraps and a Swedish skin-care system. Virtual reality relaxation and fitness equipment is also available. Gourmet cuisine is

served at the beautifully situated Lake View Restaurant.
74855 Country Club Drive, Palm Desert, CA 92260.
Tel: 1 760 341 1811

The Oaks at Ojai

The perfect venue if you want to lose weight and trim down. Spa diets ensure that you stick to a healthy low-calorie menu. In addition to a huge choice of fitness facilities, Ojai offers evening lectures on a variety of health and fitness subjects and arts and crafts classes. Sports include tennis and mountain biking. There are swimming pools, saunas and whirlpools, and a gymnasium.
122 East Ojai Avenue, Ojai, CA 93023.
Tel: 1 805 646 5573

Murrieta Day Spa

Located on natural hot springs, Murrieta specialises in a wide variety of water therapies, including mineral baths, mud baths and mineral-rich body wraps. There are three mineral-water swimming pools and one Olympic-sized pool, 14 tennis courts and an 18-hole golf course. There are fitness facilities and holistic therapies.
41885 Ivy Street, Murrieta, CA 92562.
Tel: 1 909 677 8111

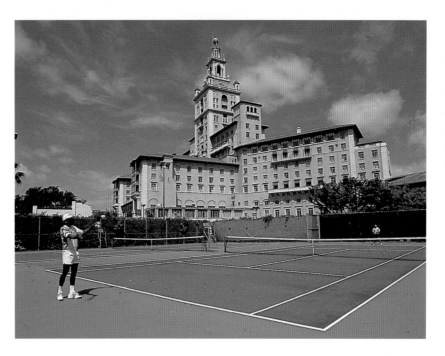

The magnificent Biltmore Hotel, Florida (see page 116), has tennis courts, a golf course, and a spa that specialises in pampering of every kind.

Colorado
The Peaks at Telluride

Set in the rugged landscape of Colorado, The Peaks offers a range of treatments from ten kinds of facials, herbal wraps and mud baths to therapeutic mineral baths and saunas. Also includes an active fitness programme of swimming, rafting, indoor climbing, squash and raquetball.
136 Country Club Drive, Telluride, CO 81435.
Tel: 1 970 728 6800

Gold Lake Mountain Resort and Spa

Situated high in the mountains, Gold Lake provides a wonderful natural environment to relax in. It offers a wide range of treatments such as Swedish massage, shiatsu, reiki, thalassotherapy, aromatherapy, craniosacral and polarity therapy, and reflexology. Other activities include canoeing, kayaking, sailing, mountain biking and volleyball. The food is organically grown and comprises whole grains and free-range animal products when possible.
3371 Gold Lake Road, Ward, CO 80481
Tel: 1 303 459 3544

Florida
Doral Saturnia spa

Exquisitely laid out with Roman arches and cascading fountains, the Doral Saturnia is a perfect place to relax and get fit. Facilities include fully equipped fitness studios, outdoor and indoor swimming pools, a wide array of water treatments and a fabulous beauty salon, the Institute de Saturnia, which boasts exclusive Italian beauty products. Cuisine comprises gourmet dishes and an exclusive spa menu.
8755 Northwest 36th Street, Miami, FL 33178.
Tel: 1 800 331 7768

Whirlpool baths and other water therapies are among the huge selection of health, fitness and beauty treatments at the Sanibel Harbour Resort, Florida.

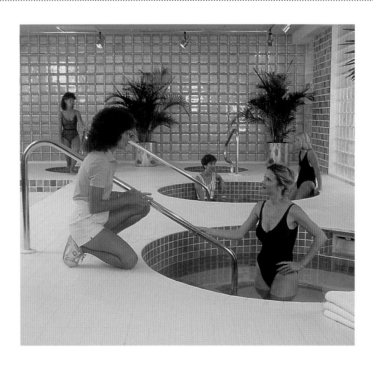

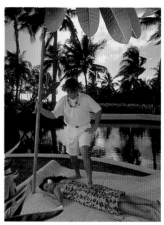

A Polynesian foot massage in a landscape of waving palm trees and limpid water is one of the delights of the Ihilani Resort and Spa, Hawaii.

Safety Harbor Resort & Spa

Located at Tampa Bay, Safety Harbor offers a comprehensive list of fitness, health and beauty facilities. There are daily fitness classes, steam baths, saunas, a variety of massage techniques, solariums and therapy pools. The Lancôme Skin Care Institute offers a stunning selection of beauty treatments. Cuisine includes a gourmet and a special spa menu.
105 North Bayshore Drive,
Safety Harbor, FL 34695.
Tel: 1 800 237 0155

Sanibel Harbour Resort

Located on the Florida coast, this resort is renowned for its superb health, fitness and beauty facilities. There is a huge selection of activities and treatments, including tennis, whirlpool baths, hot and cold plunge pools, Swiss showers, herbal wraps and cellulite treatments. The cuisine is excellent, and includes many delicious seafood dishes.
17260 Harbour Pointe Drive,
Fort Myers, FL 33908.
Tel: 1 941 466 4000

The Spa at the Biltmore

Located in the luxurious Biltmore Hotel in Coral Gables. Pampering health, beauty and fitness treatments include cellulite wraps, hydrotherapy, invigorating shower treatments, saunas, whirlpools, facials and massage of every description. There are tennis courts, a golf course and a fully equipped gym. The spa menu is superb, and you can even try your hand at health food cooking classes.
1200 Anastasia Avenue,
Coral Gables, FL 33134.
Tel: 1 305 445 1926

Hawaii
Ihilani Resort and Spa

Located on the western shore of Oahui, the spa offers fitness and relaxation programmes, hydro-therapies, such as thalassotherapy, and you can play golf and swim. Four restaurants cater for all; the speciality is the light spa cuisine.
Ko Olina Resort,
92–1001 Olani Street,
Kopalu, Hawaii 96707.
Tel: 1 808 679 0079
Fax: 1 808 679 0080

New York
New Age Health Spa

A holistic retreat set in the wooded landscape of the Catskill Mountains. This spa offers just about every new-age treatment and therapy you can think of, ranging from astrological consultations to meditation and yoga. You can also choose swimming, aerobics and weight training. Other treatments include shiatsu massage, herbal wraps, mineral-water therapies and luffa bath scrubs. There is a special spa diet and nutritional consultations. Accommodation is basic and functional.
Route 55,
Neversink, NY 12765.
Tel: 1 914 985 7600

Europe

FRANCE
Biovimer, Côte d'Azur

Situated on the Baie des Anges, Nice, with views over the sea. This is the largest sea-water therapy and fitness centre in Europe. Choose from a vast array of treatments, including bubbling baths, water massage, spray showers, mud packs, sea water pools and underwater massage. Biovimer also offers beauty treatments, such as biological facelifts and anti-ageing facials. The centre also includes a gym, two swimming pools, private beach, steam baths, saunas and a variety of fitness classes.
Marina Baie des Anges, 06270 Villeneuve-Loubet.
Tel: 334 932 271 71

Helianthal, St. Jean de Luz

Helianthal is world-famous for its thalassotherapy treatments. It also provides superb cuisine, and has nutritionists on hand to offer dietary advice. The centre is fully equipped with sports and fitness facilities, and offers beauty treatments and special weight-reduction regimes.
BP 469, Place Maurice Ravel, 64504 St. Jean de Luz.
Tel: 335 59 51 51 51

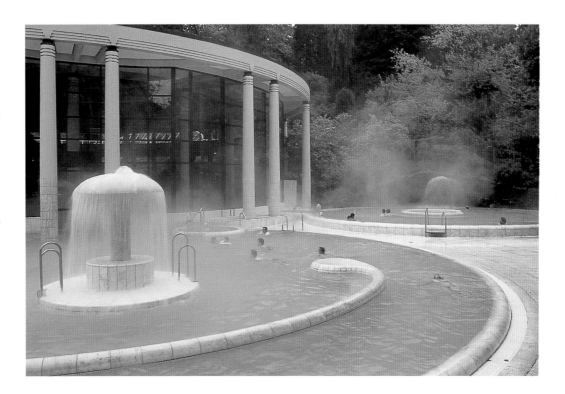

GERMANY
Caracalla Therme Hot Spring Baden-Baden

This huge complex is divided into two main areas; the ancient Roman Baths and the more modern *Friedrichbad*. The complex contains a therapy pool with water sprays and jets, and a surge channel, plus three saunas including one with coloured light therapy. Treatments are available for arthritis and circulatory disorders with thalassotherapy and massage. There is a gym, aerobics classes and sports injury specialists on site. The Caracalla is owned by the town and open to the public, with many hotels located nearby.
Römerplatz,
76530 Baden-Baden.
Tel: 49 72 21 2759 20,40

HUNGARY
Danubius Thermal Hotel, Heviz

Set in a park, this beautiful hotel overlooks Lake Heviz — one of the largest thermal lakes in the world, which has an average temperature of 34°C (93°F) in the summer and 26°C (79°F)

The hot spring at Baden-Baden in Germany, a fashionable spa town in the 19th century, continues to attract thousands of visitors.

in the winter. The hotel has its own spa, offering mud treatments, hydrotherapy, sulphur and fluoride packs, phytotherapy, dermatology and dietetic advice. The restaurant offers international, Hungarian, and dietetic menus.
H–8300 Heviz,
Kossuth L.u. 13–15.
Tel: 36 82 18 947
Fax: 36 82 18 970

ITALY
Hotel Terme di Saturnia, Grosseto
Situated at the foot of the medieval village of Saturnia in northwestern Italy and renowned for its mineral-water therapies. The thermal water surrounds the hotel — and you need to become accustomed to its distinctive sulphurous aroma! The food is excellent. The spa also has a great beauty centre.
58050 Saturnia, Grosseto.
Tel: 564 601 061
Fax: 564 601 266

SPAIN
Hotel Byblos, Mijas
Famous Andalusian health and fitness retreat which boasts two international 18-hole golf courses and offers a wide range of thalassotherapy treatments. Other amenities include sports facilities, two freshwater pools, relaxation rooms and a beauty salon.
Mijas Golf, Apt 138,
Fuengirola, Málaga.
Tel: 95 246 0250
Fax: 95 247 6783

SWITZERLAND
Le Mirador Resort and Spa, Mont Pélérin
Set in a breathtaking location, in the hills overlooking Vevey and Lake Geneva. It offers a comprehensive range of health and beauty treatments, including

Thermal waters in the historic Swiss town of Baden — named, like many spa sites, for its baths.

hydrotherapy, and a variety of therapeutic massage and cellulite-firming treatments. Also available are anti-stress treatments. Activities nearby include golf, sailing and water-skiing. The cuisine is superb (there are two restaurants), and there is a unique spa menu which incorporates cooking with essential oils.
1801 Mont Pélérin.
Tel: 21 925 1111
Fax: 21 925 1112

Hotel Maison Blanche, Leukerbad
In a spectacular mountain retreat, 1,500 metres (5,000 feet) up in the Swiss Alps, Hotel Maison Blanche has its own thermal pools, and an outdoor Jacuzzi with a mountain view. It provides a wide range of thermal treatments and a beauty salon.
3954 Leukerbad,
Tel: 27 62 11 61
Fax: 27 470 3474

Staadhof, Verenahof and Schweizerhof Hotels, Baden
Located in the traditional spa town of Baden, these hotels are all in the old quarter, close to the

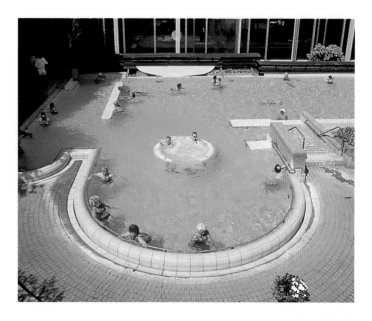

thermal centre. The hotels are renowned for their therapeutic treatments offered in a beautiful, historic setting. They include ozone therapy, and anticellulite and other beauty treatments.
Thermalkurort Baden,
Kurplatz, CH–5400 Baden.
Tel: 56 203 9393
Fax: 56 203 9394

UK
Forest Mere
Recently refurbished to create a state-of-the-art spa, Forest Mere is set in beautiful countryside. It comprises a full array of spa treatments, a beauty salon, fitness and sports facilities, a gym, two pools and a comprehensive range of alternative therapies. The

cuisine includes the choice of five-star cooking or a light spa menu.
Liphook, Hampshire GU30 7JQ.
Tel: 1428 722051

Grayshot Hall Health and Fitness Retreat
Located in beautiful countryside, the facilities are luxurious and offer a huge range of health, fitness and beauty treatments, and sports amenities. Alternative therapies include tai chi, yoga, and relaxation counselling.
Headley Road, Grayshot,
Nr. Hindhead, Surrey GU26 6JJ.
Tel: 1428 604331

Champneys Health Resort
World-famous for its health and beauty treatments, this is a luxury

resort. Therapies and activities include aromatherapy, light therapy, shiatsu and even juggling lessons. It provides five-star cuisine and a light spa menu. Wiggington, Tring, Hertfordshire HP23 6HY. Tel: 1442 291000

Stobo Castle Health Spa

An imposing Gothic castle set in lush Scottish countryside. It offers a beauty salon, an impressive array of treatments, including thalassotherapy, alternative therapies, and relaxation classes, and is fully equipped with sports and fitness facilities. Food tends to be traditional Scottish fare. Stobo Castle, Peebleshire, Scotland EH45 8NY. Tel: 1721 760249

Chewton Glen Hotel Health and Country Club

An exquisite location for a variety of health, fitness and beauty treatments. Perfect for a truly relaxing break. Superb cuisine. Christchurch Road, New Milton, Hampshire BH25 6QS. Tel: 1425 275341 Fax: 1425 272310

The Bath Spa Hotel

Set in the oldest spa town in Britain. It offers excellent spa facilities, including sauna, pool, a wide range of exercise

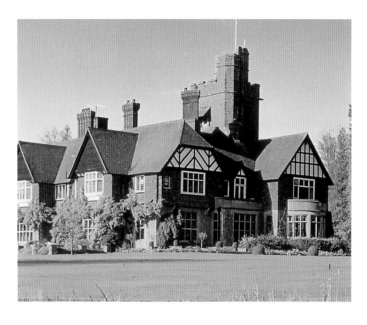

programmes, relaxing massage treatments and pampering beauty treatments. The hotel offers a fine restaurant. Sydney Road, Bath, Avon BA2 6JF. Tel: 1225 444424 Fax: 1225 444006

The Runnymede Hotel

A quaint old-world hotel offering a comprehensive range of health, beauty and spa treatments. Windsor Road, Egham, Surrey TW20 0AG. Tel: 1784 436171

Turnberry Hotel, Golf Courses and Spa

Surrounded for miles by golf courses, this Scottish hotel also offers superb spa facilities and five-star cuisine. Turnberry, Ayrshire, Scotland KA26 9LT. Tel: 1655 331000

Henlow Grange Health Farm

A Georgian mansion in calming green countryside. It offers virtually every kind of regular health and beauty treatment, has a fully equipped gym, exercise classes, and a selection of alternative therapies. Henlow, Bedfordshire SG16 6DB. Tel: 1462 811111

Ragdale Hall Health Hydro

Enjoys a lovely country location. It provides almost every

Grayshott Hall offers fine facilities and a vast choice of health and beauty therapies.

treatment you can think of, including a wide range of alternative therapies. Ragdale Village, Nr Melton Mowbray, Leicestershire, LE14 3PB. Tel: 1664 434831

Cedar Falls Health Farm

A small, secluded health farm in southwest England, which specialises in alternative therapies — from naturopathy and aromatherapy to kinesiology, iridology and reiki healing. Also offers an extensive list of beauty treatments. Bishops Lydeard, Taunton, Somerset. Tel: 1823 433233 Fax: 1823 432777

Sopwell House Hotel

Set in Hertfordshire countryside, north of London. Along with a wide range of health, fitness and beauty treatments, it features a stunning pool and fully equipped gym. Cottonmill Lane, Sopwell, St. Albans, Hertfordshire AL1 2HQ. Tel: 1727 864477 Fax: 1727 844741

Worldwide

AUSTRALIA
Hopewood Health Centre
Activities including tennis and
water aerobics. Specialities are
a cleansing food-combining
regime and therapeutic massage.
P.O. Box 38, Wallacia,
NSW 2745.
Tel: 61 2 4773 8401

**Crystal Lodge Blue
Mountains Health Retreat**
Located in the heart of the Blue
Mountains, the Lodge offers
stunning views, birdsong and
the smell of the gum trees in the
background. Relax and revive
with beauty therapies, massage
and a healing programme. For
excitement, a motorcycle ride or
joy flight are on offer.
19 Abbotsford Road,
Katoomba, NSW 2780.
Tel: 61 2 4782 5122

McCarthy Park
Choose from an extensive range
of beauty and massage
therapies or reflexology. A
rejuvenation programme focuses
on nutrition and healthy living.
There's tennis, swimming and
water aerobics for the active.
785 Berry Road,
Gidgegannup, WA 6083.
Tel: 61 8 9574 7161

*The Four Seasons Resort in Bali,
which specialises in natural herb,
clay and water therapy, and
traditional Hindu therapy.*

COSTA RICA
**El Tucan Thermae and Spa,
San Carlos**
Located in the mountains of San
Carlos, El Tucan is surrounded
by forest and set alongside the
San Rafael River, renowned for
its natural rich, volcanic, thermo-
mineral springs. El Tucan offers
health, rejuvenation, relaxation,
fitness and beauty programmes.
The sulphuric healing waters are
used to treat many ailments,
including rheumatism, arthritis
and skin disease. There is
also a therapeutic outdoor
swimming pool. Other activities
include horse-riding, walking
natural forest trails and
enjoying outdoor thermal
Jacuzzis. The hotel provides
international cuisine.
Ciudad Quesada, San Carlos.
Tel: 506 460 6000
Fax: 506 460 1692

INDONESIA
**Four Seasons Resort,
Sayan, Bali**
Nestling in the central highlands
of Bali, the spa at Sayan offers
a heavenly retreat. The emphasis
is on natural herb, botanic and
clay treatments. Specialties

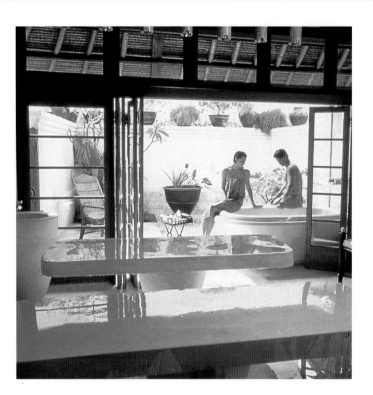

include rice and spice body
scrubs, herbal elixir massages,
and a variety of ayurvedic
(traditional Hindu therapy)
health treatments. There are also
healing water treatments, and
holistic, botanical beauty
therapies. There is a fully
equipped gym and a range of
sports and exercise facilities.
Food includes light, nutritious
Indonesian dishes.
Jimbaran,
Denpasar 80361,
Bali.
Tel: 361 701 010
Fax: 361 701 020

Javana Spa
Located on the slopes of Mount
Sarak, which is considered a
spiritual place of healing, the
guests are housed in bungalows
set among streams, waterfalls
and ponds. The spa offers a
wide range of aerobic classes,
massage and skin treatments.
More active guests can go rafting
or on guided forest hikes. Cuisine
is low-fat using vegetables and
herbs grown on the premises.
Plaza Bisnis Kemang 2,
J1 Kemang Raya No. 2,
Kemang, Jakarta 12730.
Tel: 62 21 719 8327

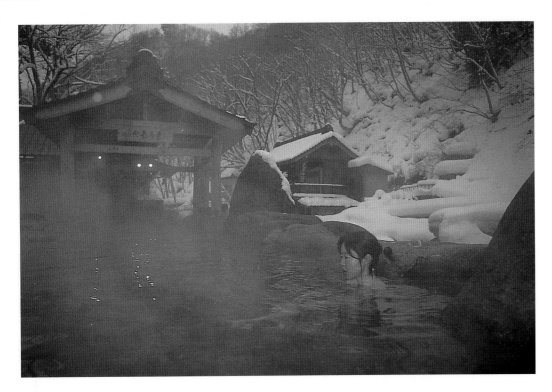

The resort of Takaragawa in Japan offers the bather the delicious sensation of wallowing in hot spring water amid the snow and ice of winter.

JAPAN
Ryokan Kannawa-En, Beppu

This is one of a number of hotels located in Beppu, a town that contains eight natural springs. Every spring has different therapeutic properties. The regime is fairly spartan and health-oriented, comprising a range of mineral-water therapies, sand baths, hot and cold water treatments, steam and mud baths. No stay is complete without exploring the exquisite surrounding countryside.

6 Kumi Kannawa Miyuki, Beppu-shi, Ohita-ken.
Tel: 81 977 66 21 11

Takaragawa Onsen

Enjoy the thermal waterfall or experience open-air baths (which are communal for women only). The alkaline water treats stiff joints and skin irritations. The menu includes river fish, mountain vegetables and hand-made noodles.
Osenkaku,
Minakarni-machi, Tone-gun, Gunma-ken 325-04
Tel: 81 278 75 21 21

NEW ZEALAND
Kim Ora Holiday and Health Resort

A peaceful, smoke-free spa set in a pine forest an hour from Nelson. Vegetarian cuisine with organically grown ingredients from the resort's garden. Gym, absailing wall, and fitness training combine with massage, hot packs and water treatments.
c/o Post Office,
Kaiteriteri,
Nelson.
Tel: 643 527 8027
Fax: 643 527 8134

Mana Retreat Centre

Established as a retreat for unwinding and reflection, the centre offers meditation, tai chi and yoga. Massage and Hellerwork is available, and there is a plunge pool, tennis and volleyball.
RD 1, Coromandel.
Tel: 647 866 8972
Fax: 647 866 8214

Hanmer Springs Thermal Reserve

This spa offers seven thermal pools and a freshwater pool. Choose from a therapeutic massage, aqua therapy/hydrotherapy, hot packs and medical baths. Gym, yoga, aerobics and also meditation.
Amuri Road, PO Box 30, Hanmer Springs.
Tel/fax: 64 3 315 7511

SOUTH AFRICA
The Hydro at Stellenbosch

Situated in the picturesque Ida's Valley, just outside historic Stellenbosch, The Hydro is surrounded by breathtaking mountain and wooded views. The natural health programme

includes lifestyle consultations, massages, hydrotherapy, steam baths, and body circulation treatments. Also available are tai chi, shiatsu, reiki, aromatherapy, thalassotherapy, and seaweed wraps. There are fitness and beauty facilities also.
PO Box 2052,
Stellenbosch,
7601 Cape.
Tel: 27 21 883 8600
Fax: 27 21 883 8390

THAILAND
Chiva-Som International Health Resort
Located by a lake, Chiva-Som resembles a little village. Accommodation is in separate bungalows. Treatments include Thai specialties, such as Thai massage and acupressure. There are extensive fitness facilities and also beauty treatments.
Petkasem Road,
Prachuap Khiri Khan 77110.
Tel: 66 32 536 536
Fax: 66 32 511 154

The Four Seasons Regent, Chiang Mai
This luxury resort in the lush countryside of northern Thailand offers a once-in-a-lifetime experience. Treatments, which are marvellously regenerating,

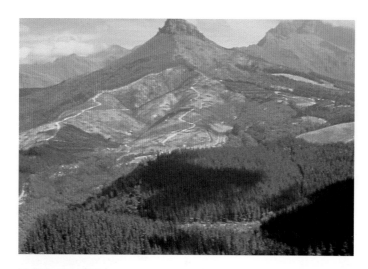

are based on the principles of Eastern philosophy. Special therapies include Thai massage, reflexology, and detoxifying herbal wraps, along with acupressure and aromatic massages with herbal and plant extracts that revitalise and rejuvenate mind and body. The food is superb — light, healthy and very Thai.
Mae Rim Samoeng Old Road,
Mae Rim, Chiang Mai 50180.
Tel: 66 53 298 181
Fax: 66 53 298 189

Oriental Hotel Spa, Bangkok
Not to be missed when in Bangkok. The spa is situated a short boat trip across the river from the main hotel. The treatments are spectacular. The

spa is pristine and the setting is tranquil. Beauty treatments are also available, comprising the spa's own luxurious line of products. You need not be a guest at the hotel to visit the spa, which is open to day-guests.
48 Oriental Ave,
Bangkok 10500.
Tel: 66 2 236 0400
Fax: 66 2 236 1937

TURKEY
Kervansaray Thermal Hotel, Bursa
Located in a luxurious five-star hotel, these spa facilities are designed to relax and pamper. The town of Bursa is renowned for its natural hot springs. Mineral-water therapies, including special rheumatism

Stunning views of forest and mountain enhance the natural therapies at South Africa's Hydro.

treatments, are the main feature of the spa. Also included are other health and beauty treatments, including massage, Turkish baths, aromatic beauty treatments, and a range of fitness facilities. The food is typically Turkish.
Cekirge Maydani,
Cekirge Bursa.
Tel: 90 224 233 9300
Fax: 90 233 9324

The Spa Hotel Colossae Thermal Pamukkale
In western Turkey, within walking distance of the ancient town of Hierapolis and the natural park of Pamukkale. The park is renowned for its white lakes, formed from lime deposits left on the mountainside by the mineral waters. The hotel contains a spa health centre staffed by a team of qualified physiotherapists and beauty specialists. Programmes include water therapy, skin-care, and anti-ageing treatments.
Karahayit, Pamukkale, Denizli.
Tel: 90 258 271 4156
Fax: 90 258 271 4250

Regeneration is the essence of the traditional Thai treatments at The Four Seasons Regent, Chiang Mai.

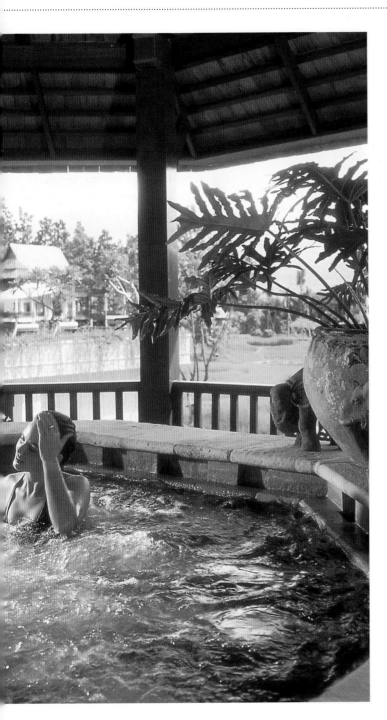

Glossary of terms

Active ingredients

The key ingredients in a product that produce a specific physiological effect.

Alkalis

Substances with a pH above 7 (strong alkalis are corrosive — for example caustic soda).

Alkaloids

Plant substances which have a pharmacological effect.

Alkyloamides

A group of ingredients (cocamide, DEA, MEA, MIPA), which are used in shampoos and body cleansers. They have thickening, gelling, emulsifying properties.

Allantoin

A natural derivative of comfrey, which has soothing properties and is often included in moisturisers.

Alpha hydroxy acids (AHAs)

A generic term describing a range of simple, naturally occurring acids derived from milk, sugar cane and fruits. All have a mild exfoliant effect, which gently rids the skin of dead cells and makes it appear smoother and less lined immediately after application.

Amino acids

A set of compounds that make up proteins. Some are produced naturally by the body — for example arginine, cystine and taurine; others, such as leucine, histidine and lysine, are not. There are 22 chief amino acids that are essential for good health.

Ammonium lauryl sulphate

A synthetic detergent. It is a foaming and cleansing agent derived from the salt of sulphated lauryl alcohol.

Antibacterial

Any substance that inhibits the growth of bacteria — for example some essential oils. Also known as antimicrobial.

Antioxidants

Vitamins such as A, C and E that neutralise the effect of free radicals. Free radicals are unstable, oxidised cells — caused by factors such as UV light, pollution and smoking — which disrupt the mechanism of cell repair.

Astringent
A substance that causes the constriction of pores.

Azulene
The anti-inflammatory compound found in camomile flowers.

Benzaldehyde
The main component of almond oil. Can cause allergies.

Benzene
A petrochemical solvent found in many cosmetics. Can be highly toxic.

Benzoic acid
An antimicrobial used in cosmetics to stop bacteria growing.

Botanical extract
A substance extracted from plants.

Calcium carbonate
A naturally occurring white calcium salt found in limestone and chalk.

Ceramides
Moisture-retaining substances found between skin cells in the upper layers of the skin.

Cellulose
A synthetic gum used as a stabiliser and thickener.

Chlorophyll
The green pigment in plants. Essential for photosynthesis.

Cocamide DEA
A surfactant (cleanser) derived from coconut oil.

Collagen
A body protein found in all connective tissues. It deteriorates with age and causes wrinkles to appear.

Detergent
A chemical cleansing agent (may be derived from petroleum or vegetable oils).

Elastin
A protein of elastic tissue, present in the skin, ligaments and arterial walls.

Emollient
A moisturising substance which prevents moisture loss from the skin.

Emulsifier
A substance that holds oil in water or water in oil (the two substances that notoriously do not mix) — for example borax, beeswax. Used in the manufacture of creams and lotions.

Essential fatty acid
The body cannot produce fatty acids but they are vital for good health — for example linoleic acid. Found in some oils, such as evening primrose oil.

Ester
An acid derivative (usually smells fruity).

Fuller's earth
A talc-like clay which draws out impurities from the skin.

Fixative
A substance that slows down evaporation of ingredients — for example in fragrances. Includes some essential oils.

Gelatin
A thickener made from the bones and hides of animals.

Glucose glutamate
A conditioning and moisturising agent derived from glucose and glutanic acid.

Glyceryl stearate
An emulsifying and moisturising agent produced from glycerol and stearic acid.

Humectant
A moisturising substance that reduces moisture loss from the surface of the skin.

Hypoallergenic
A substance that will not cause skin irritation.

Infusion
A solution made by adding herbs or plant matter to boiling water and left to steep or brew — normally for 10 minutes.

Iron oxide
A substance widely used as a pigment in cosmetics.

Kaolin
A white powdery clay, used in face powders and masks. Absorbs oils.

Keratin
A substance found in hair and nails.

Lanolin
A highly emollient substance derived from sheep's wool fat.

Lecithin
A natural emulsifier derived from soya oil.

Lipids
Naturally occurring fats in the skin.

Lauric acid
A fatty acid found in laurel and coconut oil.

Liposomes
Microscopic artificial sacs. Used to convey substances into cells in the skin. An ingredient of moisturisers.

Mineral oil
A by-product of petroleum. Not easily absorbed by the skin, and can cause irritation.

Oleic acid
An emollient derived from animal or vegetable fats. Can cause irritation.

Oxidation
A chemical reaction which causes oils and fats to go rancid.

Pantothenic acid (B5)
A B-complex, water-soluble vitamin used in hair products for its moisturising properties.

Parabens
Natural esters used as preservatives. Can be synthetically reproduced to stop bacterial growth in a product.

Paraffin wax
A white, waxy, odourless substance derived from petrochemicals. Used as a moisturiser.

PABA
A water-soluble acid (para-aminobenzoic acid) derived from B vitamins. Found in sunscreens.

Pectin
A thickener derived from fruit rinds.

PEG derivatives
Used as humectants and moisturising agents.

Phytotherapy
The therapeutic use of plants and herbs.

Polymer
The combination of many small molecules.

Preservative
A substance that inhibits bacterial and fungal growth. Used to prolong the life of cosmetics and personal care products.

Propylene glycol
A synthetically produced odourless liquid, used as a solvent in perfumes and a humectant in cosmetics.

Retinoids
Derivatives of vitamin A, used in anti-ageing and acne treatments.

Salicylic acid
A naturally occurring fruit acid.

Saponification
The reaction of a fat or oil with a strong base — such as caustic soda — used in making soap.

Saponins
Sugar-based substances which occur naturally in some plants — for example soapwort. Used for their foaming and cleansing properties.

Shellac
A resinous substance secreted by insects. Used as a binder in hair spray.

Silicone
A group of oils derived from the mineral silica.

Sodium carbonate
Washing soda, used in detergents.

Sodium chloride
Common salt.

Sodium hydroxide
Caustic soda. Used in the manufacture of soap.

Sodium lauryl sulphate
A synthetic detergent. It is one of the few biodegradable detergents.

Stearic acid
A fatty acid derived from animal and vegetable fats. Used as an emulsifier.

Tallow
Fat obtained from animal fatty tissue (for example sheep), used to make soaps and emulsifiers.

Tannins
Astringent substances found in plants.

Tincture
Alcohol and water used to derive plant extracts.

Tocopherol
A vitamin-E derivative, used as an antioxidant in cosmetics.

Viscosity
A term that describes how sticky or fluid a product is.

Xanthum gum
Gum derived from corn sugar, used as a thickener and stabiliser.

Zinc oxide
Natural mineral powder, used in cosmetics. A natural sunscreen.

Zinc pyrithione
A synthetic anti-dandruff ingredient in shampoos. Can irritate the skin.

Index

**Page numbers in italics
refer to illustrations**

Credits

Quarto Publishing plc would like to thank and acknowledge the following for pictures used in this book.

Hotel Verenahof: 118; The Biltmore Hotel: 15; Canyon Ranch: 113; Corbis UK Ltd: 10 tr; e. t. archive: 9, 62 b & t, 63, 87; Four Seasons Resort Bali, at Jimbaran Bay: 108 tl, 120; Chris Fairclough: 76 bl; Getty Images: 8 bl, 32 br, 33, 46 b, 46 t, 86 b; Eva Gizowska: 7; Golden Door Spa: 114 l; Grayshott Hall: 119; The Hydro at Stellenbosch: 122; Image Bank: 11, 32 bl, 86 t; Image Select: 8 br; Ihilani Resort and Spa: 116 r; J L Mott Iron Works: 10 b; Michael Manuel/The Greenhouse: 109 t; Kevin Orpin/The Regent Resort Chiang Mai: 123; Pictor International: 76 br; The Peaks Resort & Spa: 114 r; Grand Lido Sans Souci/Superclubs: 112; Sanibel Harbour Resort & Spa: 110, 116 l; The Stockmarket Photo Agency Inc: 117, 121; Visual Arts Library: 77; World Pictures: 47. All other photographs are the copyright of Quarto Publishing plc.

While every effort has been made to contact all copyright holders, Quarto would like to apologize for any omissions.

The author and Quarto Publishing plc would like to thank The Bath Spa Hotel, Bath, England, for kindly allowing us to use the facilities of the "Laurels Health and Leisure Spa" for photography. Quarto would also like to thank the models for their cooperation and CPHart, Newnham Terrace, Hercules Road, London SE1 7DR, for supplying the bath and fittings used in photography.

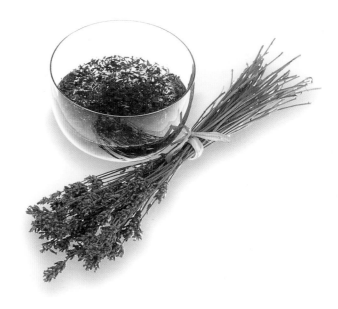